健康评估技能操作指导
（中英双语）

A MANUAL OF HEALTH ASSESSMENT SKILLS
（CHINESE-ENGLISH EDITION）

王克芳　主审

李　静　主编

U0238941

山东大学出版社
SHANDONG UNIVERSITY PRESS
·济南·

图书在版编目(CIP)数据

健康评估技能操作指导:汉英对照/李静主编.—
济南:山东大学出版社,2022.4
ISBN 978-7-5607-7428-2

Ⅰ.①健… Ⅱ.①李… Ⅲ.①健康—评估—汉、英
Ⅳ.①R471

中国版本图书馆 CIP 数据核字(2022)第 058852 号

策划编辑　徐　翔
责任编辑　毕文霞
文案编辑　毕玉璇
封面设计　王秋忆

出版发行　山东大学出版社
社　　址　山东省济南市山大南路 20 号
邮政编码　250100
发行热线　(0531)88363008
经　　销　新华书店
印　　刷　山东蓝海文化科技有限责任公司
规　　格　720 毫米×1000 毫米　1/16
　　　　　7 印张　150 千字
版　　次　2022 年 4 月第 1 版
印　　次　2022 年 4 月第 1 次印刷
定　　价　58.00 元

《健康评估技能操作指导》
（中英双语）
A MANUAL OF HEALTH ASSESSMENT SKILLS
（CHINESE-ENGLISH EDITION）
编委会名单

主　审　　王克芳

主　编　　李　静

副主编　　贾　愚　郭玉芳　刘　丽

编　者　　（以姓氏笔画为序）

　　　　　刘　丽　北京中医药大学护理学院

　　　　　李玉丽　山东大学护理与康复学院

　　　　　李　静　山东大学护理与康复学院

　　　　　赵倩倩　南方医科大学护理学院

　　　　　战同霞　潍坊医学院护理学院

　　　　　郭玉芳　山东大学护理与康复学院

　　　　　贾　愚　山东大学护理与康复学院

示　教　　李　静　贾　愚

配　音　　郭玉芳（中文配音）　贾　愚（英文配音）

字　幕　　郭平

剪　辑　　郭平

秘　书　　郭玉芳　山东大学护理与康复学院

序

高等教育国际化作为世界高等教育发展的重要趋势,被各国置于教育政策的核心位置。来华留学生教育和中外合作办学是我国高等教育国际化发展的重要形式。为满足全球化的需要,各护理院校陆续开展留学生教育和中外合作办学,以培养具有国际意识、具备国际交往和国际竞争能力的高素质护理人才。山东大学护理与康复学院积极推动护理教育国际化,于2017年开始招收护理学专业本科来华留学生,在该项目实施过程中,基于全英语和双语教学的需要,健康评估课程组教师联合姊妹院校教师编写了此教材。

此教材英语表达专业、规范,中文表达精练,有助于读者准确理解英文内容。书中按照从头到脚的顺序介绍了健康评估课程中所涉及的重要操作技能,最后通过案例的形式引导学生将健康评估技能用于发现受检者的健康问题,符合整体护理的工作理念和方法。本教材清晰、详细地阐述了各项技能操作方法,并说明了其阳性体征的临床意义,为读者解难释疑;每项操作之后附注英语生词,可帮助读者掌握单词的含义,便于理解内容。中、英文两套配音的操作视频,提高了教材的直观性,扩大了教材的适用群体。另外,英文配音版本添加了英语字幕,有助于读者更好地理解和掌握其中含义。

此教材体现了国际护理教育理念与全英语及双语教学的特点,既可用于来华留学生教学和护理学专业双语(全英文)教学,又可作为护理学专业学生英语能力训练的辅助教材,适合护理学专业学生、留学生、在职医护人员和有志于从事国际护理工作的护理人员阅读。这是一本系统、全面的优秀双语教材,特向广大护理工作者和护理专业学生推荐。

山东大学护理与康复学院院长 王克芳

2022 年 3 月

前　言

　　健康评估实践涉及通过评估发现受检者的健康问题,既包括操作技能,又包括受检者与医务人员之间的沟通与合作等,在整个护理学专业教育中占据重要地位。随着护理教育国际化,护理人才交流国际化,护士岗位国际化,我国各护理院校陆续开展了来华留学生教育,开设了中外合作护理学专业。为满足护理学专业来华留学生教学与双语及全英文教学的需求,我们在尊重英语国家语言习惯的基础上,结合我国护理操作流程,编写了《健康评估技能操作指导》(中英双语)。

　　本教材在培养学生健康评估操作能力的同时,融入了国外先进的护理教育理念,充分尊重受检者自尊和隐私,体现了人文关怀,强调了临床思维的重要性以及评估技能在护理工作中的应用,以发现受检者存在的健康问题,引导学生从单纯地获得技能转向具有临床思维、能够提供人性化的以人为中心的服务,培养既能适应国内医疗机构的工作环境,又能适应外资医院或国外医疗机构的工作环境,具有较强国际竞争力的高素质国际化护理人才。

　　配套视频旨在更好地帮助学生进行健康评估课程操作技能的学习。

　　在此教材出版之际,我要感谢山东大学护理与康复学院的支持,感谢课程组老师辛勤的付出和对于视频拍摄的大力协助,感谢为此教材的出版付出辛勤努力的全体成员,最后还要感谢家人给予我的理解和支持!

1

　　由于编者水平及各方面条件的限制，书中难免有不当及疏漏之处，敬请护理同仁及同学们不吝指正，使这本教材可以不断得到完善。

李静

2022 年 3 月

CONTENTS
目　录

Assessment Skill 1
Basic Assessment Skills

评估技能 1
基本评估技能

1-1　Inspection

Inspection is a diagnostic method in which an examiner uses eyes to observe an examinee's whole body or regional parts. It can be divided into whole body inspection and local inspection.

Whole body inspection can be applied in assessing the patient's general condition and signs，such as age，development，nutrition，consciousness，mental status，complexion，facial expression，body position，pose，gait，etc.

Local inspection can help examiners to discover changes in different parts of the body of the examinee，such as the skin，mucosa，eyes，ears，etc.

1-1　视诊

视诊是评估者通过视觉了解受检者全身或局部状态有无异常的检查方法，可以分为全身视诊和局部视诊。

全身视诊可以用于评估受检者一般状况和体征，如年龄、生长发育、营养、意识状态、心理状况、面容、表情、体位、姿势和步态等。

局部视诊可以帮助评估者了解受检者身体不同部位的改变，如皮肤、黏膜、眼睛、耳朵等。

1-2　Palpation

Palpation is one of the basic skills of physical assessment and can be applied in a variety of clinical settings. During abdominal palpation, the examinee should bend his/her knees and lie down face-up to fully relax the abdominal muscles. Fingertip and the palmar side of the metacarpophalangeal joint are most sensitive in tactile sense, which are usually used in palpation. Palpation can be divided into light and deep palpation.

1-2-1　Light Palpation

During the light palpation, fingers are held together, the ulnar side of finger pulps, instead of the fingertip, are put on the site of palpation. By moving the metacarpophalangeal joint and wrist in synchrony, we lightly palpate with a spinning or sliding motion. The depth of light palpation is around 1-2 cm. After palpation of one site, the hand should be lifted off the skin and moved to the next site.

Light palpation usually causes a little pain, if any, nor does it cause tension of the muscle. Therefore, it is useful in determination of tenderness, resistance, pulsation, mass or enlarged organs.

1-2　触诊

触诊是身体评估的基本技能之一,可以用在多种临床情况。腹部触诊时,受检者采取屈膝仰卧位,以充分放松腹肌。指尖和掌指关节掌侧触觉最敏感,是触诊常用的部位。触诊分为浅触诊和深触诊。

1-2-1　浅部触诊法

在腹部进行浅部触诊时,受检者取屈膝仰卧位,检查者手指并拢,将手指掌面而不是指尖放在触诊部位,利用掌指关节和腕关节的协同动作以旋转或滑动的方式轻压触摸,可触及的深度为1～2 cm。一个部位触诊结束后,手要离开皮肤,然后移到另一个部位。

浅触诊通常会引起轻微疼痛,但不会引起肌肉紧张。因此,浅触诊可用于检查腹部有无压痛、抵抗感、搏动感、包块或某些肿大的脏器。

QR code 1-2-1　Light palpation

二维码 1-2-1　浅触诊

1-2-2　Deep Palpation

During the deep palpation，the examiner can use one hand or stack both hands together. We slowly increase the depth and pressure to meet the purpose of deep palpation. The depth of palpation often exceeds 2 cm，reaches 4-5 cm. Deep palpation is used to inspect and evaluate abdominal lesions and organs. According to different goals and methods，deep palpation can be categorized into the following three types.

1-2-2-1　Deep slipping palpation：Before the examination, tell the examinee to calmly breathe through his/her mouth or have a conversation to distract his/her attention. The examinee lies in supine position with knees bent. This could relax the abdominal muscles. The examiner then adduct the index，middle and ring fingers and begin to palpate from the surface of the abdomen to deeper organs or masses. The examiner needs to move in four directions after feeling a mass. This method is used for palpation of deep masses and intestinal lesions.

1-2-2　深部触诊法

用一手或两手重叠，由浅入深，逐步施加压力以达深部，可触及的深度多在 2 cm 以上，可达 4～5 cm。深部触诊法主要用以检查腹腔内的病变和脏器的情况。根据检查目的与手法的不同，深部触诊可分为以下三种。

1-2-2-1　深部滑行触诊法：检查时，嘱患者屈膝仰卧位，张口呼吸，尽量放松腹肌，可以与患者交谈以转移其注意力，以并拢的 2、3、4 指末端逐渐触向腹腔脏器或包块，并在其上做上下左右滑动触摸，常用于腹腔深部包块和胃肠病变的检查。

QR code 1-2-2-1　Deep slipping palpation

1-2-2-2　Bimanual palpation：The examiner adducts the middle three fingers of the right hand while using the left hand to hold up the mass from the back. The mass is then lifted between the examiner's hands and is closer to body surface. In cooperation with abdominal breathing, bimanual palpation can be used for examining the liver，spleen，kidneys and visceral masses.

QR code 1-2-2-2　Bimanual palpation

1-2-2-3　Deep press palpation：This method requires press two or three fingers deeply into the desired site over 2 cm or even 4-5 cm in the abdomen. It is used to detect lesions deep within the abdomen or determine the site of tenderness，such as McBurney's point，Murphy's sign. When checking for rebound tenderness，press the fingers deeply and stay still for 2-3 s，then quickly withdraw the fingers to see if the examinee feels more pain or expresses a painful complexion.

二维码 1-2-2-1　深部滑行触诊

1-2-2-2　双手触诊法：护士将右手并拢的中间三指平置于腹壁上，左手置于被检查脏器或包块的后部，向右手方向托起，以固定脏器或包块，使其更接近体表配合右手触诊，与腹式呼吸配合，常用于肝、脾、肾及脏器肿物的触诊。

二维码 1-2-2-2　双手触诊

1-2-2-3　深压触诊法：这种方法需要用 2～3 个手指深压至被检部位 2 cm 以上，可达 4～5 cm，以探测腹腔深在病变的部位或确定腹部压痛点，如阑尾压痛点、胆囊压痛点等。检查反跳痛则是在手指深压的基础上稍停 2～3 秒，迅速将手抬起，同时询问患者有无疼痛加剧或观察其面部有无痛苦表情。

QR code 1-2-2-3　Deep press palpation

二维码 1-2-2-3　深压触诊法

1-3　Percussion

Percussion is to strike the examined part of the examinee's body using examiner's fingers or palm. According to the quality of the sound obtained，the underlying disease will be determined.

Percussion is particularly important to examine the chest and abdomen. It will be discussed in later chapters.

According to different purposes and methods，percussion can be divided into direct and indirect percussion.

1-3-1　Direct Percussion

In direct percussion，the examiner directly taps the examined part with the palm of the right fingers. According to the resonating sound and the vibration sense，the pathological changes will be verified.

1-3-2　Indirect Percussion

Indirect percussion is a percussion method commonly used under clinical settings. It includes finger percussion and fist percussion.

1-3　叩诊

叩诊是指用手指叩击或手掌拍击受检部位的表面,使之震动产生音响,根据其震动和音响特点,判断受检部位的脏器有无异常的检查方法。

叩诊在胸腹部的检查中尤为重要,将在后续的章节中讨论。

根据不同的叩诊目的和手法,可将其分为直接叩诊法和间接叩诊法。

1-3-1　直接叩诊法

在直接叩诊中,评估者用右手指的掌面拍击被检查部位,根据拍击的反响和指下的震动感,判断病变情况。

1-3-2　间接叩诊法

间接叩诊法是临床常用的叩诊方法,分为指指叩诊和捶叩诊。

Finger percussion: The examiner places the middle finger (also called the pleximeter finger) of the left hand on the site of percussion, while hyperextends other fingers to avoid contacting with the examinee's body surface, which would influence the resonance. The fingers of the right hand are flexed naturally. The examiner uses the top of the middle finger to strike the proximal or distal interphalangeal joint of the pleximeter finger of the left hand, which is closely placed on the percussion site and sensitive to resonance. The direction of the striking motion should be perpendicular to the body surface of the examined site. The motion of percussion should be oriented by the movement of the wrist and metacarpophalangeal joint, while not the elbow or shoulder joint. The striking movement should be quick, agile and flexible. The middle finger of right hand should be elevated immediately after percussion to avoid affecting the identification of percussion sound. Two or three taps can be made at each percussion site, if needed, additional percussion can be made to assist in diagnosis. Continuous striking of the same site should be avoided because of the difficulty in discerning the quality of the note. During the process of percussion, when the second knuckle of the left middle finger moves, it should be lifted and be away from the skin.

指指叩诊:评估者将左手中指作为板指放在被叩诊部位,其余手指翘起以免与胸壁接触而影响声音的传导。右手手指自然弯曲,评估者用中指指端叩击左手中指第二指关节处或第二节指骨远端,该关节紧靠叩诊部位,对共振敏感。叩击运动的方向应垂直于被检查部位的体表。叩诊的动作应以腕关节和掌指关节的动作为主,肘关节或肩关节不参与运动。叩击动作要迅速、灵活和富有弹性,每次连续叩击2～3次,必要时可再连续叩击2～3次,以协助诊断。叩击后应立即抬起右手中指,以免影响叩击声音的辨别。应避免连续敲击同一部位影响叩击音的质量。叩诊过程中,左手中指第二指节移动时,应抬起并离开皮肤,不可连同皮肤一起移动。

Fist percussion：In determining pain on percussion of the liver or renal span, the examiner can place the palm of the left hand on the desired site while making a fist with the right hand. Strike the back of the left hand with the ulnar side of the fist to evaluate the potential pain.

QR code 1-3-2　Indirect percussion

捶叩诊:在确定肝或肾区叩击痛时,评估者可以将左手的手掌放在所叩诊的位置,同时用右手握拳,用拳头的尺侧叩击左手的背部,以评估潜在的疼痛感。

二维码 1-3-2　间接叩诊法

1-4　Auscultation

Auscultation is the process that the examiner determines the presence of disease by the sound produced in the examinee's different parts of body. It is especially important in cardiac and pulmonary illnesses.

Auscultation includes direct and indirect auscultation.

1-4-1　Direct Auscultation

Direct auscultation is directly attaching one's ear to the site to examine. The sound obtained is usually very weak. This method is only used during emergencies or other special circumstances.

1-4-2　Indirect Auscultation

Indirect auscultation is a method of auscultation with the help of a stethoscope. The

1-4　听诊

听诊是评估者以听觉听取发自受检者身体各部的声音,以判断其有无疾病的检查方法,在心脏和肺脏疾病中尤为重要。

听诊包括直接听诊和间接听诊。

1-4-1　直接听诊

直接听诊是将耳直接贴于受检部位体表进行听诊的方法,该方法所能听到的体内声音微弱,仅用于紧急和特殊情况。

1-4-2　间接听诊

间接听诊为借助听诊器进行听诊的方法。听诊

stethoscope is composed of an earpiece, a chestpiece and tubing. The chestpiece can be divided into two types: the bell and the diaphragm. During auscultation, the earpiece should bend in the direction that follows the direction of the ear canal, inwards and forwards. The bell is designed for hearing sounds with a low pitch, such as the murmur of mitral stenosis. The diaphragm is used to auscultate high pitched sounds such as the murmur of aortic insufficiency, breath sounds and bowel sounds. During auscultation, the environment should be quiet and the room temperature should be suitable, so as to avoid the interference of ambient noise and the additional sound caused by muscle tremor due to coldness. The stethoscope body part is close to the skin and should be carried out in order during auscultation. When moving, the stethoscope body part should be lifted away from the skin.

器由耳件、体件和软管三部分组成,体件有钟型和膜型两种。听诊时,耳件弯曲方向顺应耳道的方向,向内前方向。钟型体件适于听取低调的声音,如二尖瓣狭窄的舒张期隆隆样杂音;膜型体件适于听取高调的声音,如主动脉瓣关闭不全的杂音、呼吸音、肠鸣音等。听诊时,要环境安静、室温适宜,避免因环境噪音及因寒冷所致肌束震颤产生的附加音的干扰。听诊器体件紧贴听诊部位的皮肤,按照顺序进行听诊。移动时,听诊器体件应离开皮肤。

QR code 1-4-2　Indirect auscultation

二维码 1-4-2　间接听诊法

Words and Expressions

adduct　*v.* 使内收

agile　*adj.* 敏捷的,灵活的

auscultation　*n.* 听诊

dullness　　*n*.浊音

flatness　　*n*.实音

inspection　　*n*.视诊

knuckle　　*n*.关节,指关节 *v*.用指关节打

metacarpophalangeal　　*adj*.掌指的

mitral stenosis　　二尖瓣狭窄

murmur　　*n*.杂音

palm　　*n*.手掌,手心

palpation　　*n*.触诊

percussion　　*n*.叩诊

perpendicular　　*adj*.垂直的

pleximeter finger　　板指

resistance　　*n*.反对,抵抗,反抗

resonance　　*n*.清音

stethoscope　　*n*.听诊器

synchrony　　*n*.同步,同步性,共时

tactile　　*adj*.触觉的,有触觉的,能触知的

tender　　*adj*.和善的,温柔的,疼痛的,触痛的

tympany　　*n*.鼓音

ulnar　　*adj*.尺骨(近尺、尺侧)的

Assessment Skill 2
Superficial Lymph Node Assessment

评估技能 2
浅表淋巴结评估

Lymph nodes distribute in the whole body, only superficial lymph nodes can be found by general assessment. The superficial lymph nodes of healthy people are very small, 0.2- 0.5 cm in diameter, soft in texture, smooth in surface, good in movement and no tenderness. Lymph nodes enlargement may occur in lymphadenitis or malignant tumor.

The inspection methods of lymph nodes include inspection and palpation, with palpation as the main method. During palpation, a sitting position for the examinee is preferred. The examiner puts the index finger, middle finger, and ring finger close to the site of examination, from the shallow to the deep site of local lymph nodes by slipping palpation, and palpates the front of the ear, the back of the ear, the suboccipital area, submandibular area, submental

人的身体遍布淋巴结，但是，只有浅表淋巴结才能在一般检查中被检查到。健康人浅表淋巴结很小，直径0.2~0.5 cm，质地柔软、表面光滑、活动良好、无压痛。淋巴结炎、恶性肿瘤淋巴结转移等可出现淋巴结肿大。

淋巴结的评估方法包括视诊和触诊，以触诊为主。触诊时，受检者取坐位，评估者以并拢的示、中、环三指紧贴检查部位，由浅入深，以指腹按压皮肤与皮下组织之间进行滑动触诊，触诊顺序为耳前、耳后、枕骨下区、颌下区、颏下区、颈前三角、颈后三角、锁骨上

area，anterior cervical triangle，posterior cervical triangle， supraclavicular fossa， axillary， upper trochlear and inguinal lymph nodes.

The examinee is either in a standing position or sitting position. The sequence of palpating axillary lymph nodes is the top，the inside wall，the anterior wall，the posterior wall and the outside wall. When palpating the inguinal lymph nodes，a supine position is required for the examinee with bent hip joint and knee joint. Palpate the horizontal group first，then the vertical group.

When checking the lymph nodes，the local skin muscles should be relaxed and fingers should be close to the site of examination palpate from the shallow to the deep site of local lymph nodes by slipping palpation.

When touching the enlarged lymph nodes，the examiner should pay attention to the location， size， numbers， hardness， tenderness， mobility， clear boundary， and local skin redness，scar，fistula，etc. At the same time，look for the primary lesions which would cause lymph nodes enlargement.

窝、腋窝、滑车上和腹股沟淋巴结。

腋窝淋巴结检查时受检者取站立位或坐位。腋窝淋巴结的触诊顺序是顶、内、前、后、外。腹股沟淋巴结触诊时受检者取仰卧位，屈膝屈髋，分别触诊水平群和垂直群。

检查淋巴结时应使局部皮肤肌肉松驰，手指紧贴检查部位，由浅入深进行滑动触诊。

触及肿大的淋巴结时应注意其部位、大小、数目、硬度、有无压痛、活动度、界限是否清楚，以及局部皮肤有无红肿、疤痕、瘘管等。同时寻找引起淋巴结肿大的原发病灶。

QR code2　Superficial lymph nodes palpation

二维码 2　浅表淋巴结触诊

Words and Expressions

anterior cervical triangle　颈前三角

axillary　*n.* 腋窝

fistula　*n.* 瘘,瘘管

inguinal　*adj.* 腹股沟的

inguinal lymph nodes　腹股沟淋巴结

lymphadenitis　*n.* 淋巴结炎

lymph node　淋巴结

malignant　*adj.* 恶性的,恶意的

posterior cervical triangle　颈后三角

submandibular area　颌下区

submental area　颏下区

sub-occipital area　枕骨下区

supraclavicular fossa　锁骨上窝

texture　*n.* 质地

upper trochlear lymph nodes　滑车上淋巴结

Assessment Skill 3
Eye Assessment

评估技能 3
眼睛评估

3-1 Conjunctiva Assessment

The examiner asks the examinee to look up and places both thumbs on the middle of the lower eyelids, then pulls the eyelid margins downward to observe the lower eyelid conjunctiva, fornix conjunctiva, bulbar conjunctiva and sclera.

The examiner asks the examinee to look down and pinches the edge of the middle and outer 1/3 of the right upper eyelid with the left index finger and thumb. The examiner gently pulls it forward and then presses it down with the index finger, and cooperates with the thumb to twist the edge of the eyelid upward. Flip the upper eyelid. Observe the eyelid conjunctiva and fornix conjunctiva. Lift the skin of the upper eyelid to turn the eyelid

3-1 眼结膜评估

评估者嘱受检者眼睛向上看,将双手拇指置于其下眼睑中部,同时向下牵拉睑缘,观察下眼睑结膜、穹隆结膜、球结膜及巩膜。

评估者嘱受检者眼睛向下看,用左手示指和拇指捏住其右上眼睑中外1/3交界处的边缘,轻轻向前牵拉,然后示指向下压,并与拇指配合,将睑缘向上捻转,翻转上眼睑,观察眼睑结膜和穹隆结膜。提起上眼睑皮肤,使眼睑翻转复原。按同样方法检查左上

over and to recover. Check the other eyelid in the same way. When turning the eyelid，be gentle and careful.

眼睑。翻转眼睑时,力度要适中,动作要轻柔。

QR code 3-1　Conjunctiva assessment

二维码 3-1　眼结膜评估

3-2　Eyeballs Movement

3-2　眼球运动

The aim of binocular movement assessment is mainly to understand the coordination of the eye movement and the intensity of the movement function of the eyes.

The examiner extends his/her right arm and erects the index finger about 30-40 cm away from the examinee's eyes. The examinee is asked to keep his/her eyes on the moving finger of the examiner and is not allowed to turn his/her head. The index finger moves in six directions：left，upper left，lower left，right，upper right，lower right. Eyeballs movement disorders and nystagmus could be determined according to the abnormal movement of the eyeballs.

双眼运动的评估主要是为了了解眼球运动的协调性和运动功能的强弱程度。

评估者伸右臂,竖食指,置于距受检者眼前30～40 cm处,嘱受检者注视手指的移动,并告之勿转动头部,食指按左、左上、左下、右、右上、右下,共 6 个方向进行移动,观察受检者有无眼球运动障碍和眼球震颤。

QR code 3-2　Eyeballs movement

二维码 3-2　眼球运动

3-3　Pupillary Light Reflex

During the process of pupil assessment, the examiner should pay attention to the shape, size, and position of the pupil; whether the two pupils are equally round or same in size; light and convergence reflex, etc. Light reflection includes direct light reflection and indirect light reflection.

In direct light reflection, the examiner can use a flashlight to illuminate the pupil directly and observe its dynamic response. Normally, the pupils will constrict when the eyes are exposed to the light and will recover when the light is removed. In the indirect reflection, exposing to light in one eye results in the constriction of the pupil of the opposite eye.

Take a flashlight and check the light reflection after focusing. The flashlight moves from the outside to the inside to directly illuminate the left pupil, and observe whether the pupil shrinks. After removing the light, keep the right eye out of light by hand and then illuminate the left pupil directly with the flashlight again to observe the dynamic response of the right pupil. Check the right side in the same way.

If the pupillary light reflex is sluggish or absent, the examinee may be in a coma.

3-3　瞳孔对光反射

瞳孔检查时应注意瞳孔的形状、大小、位置,双侧瞳孔是否等圆、等大,对光反射及集合反射等。对光反射分为直接对光反射和间接对光反射。

直接对光反射,通常用手电筒直接照射瞳孔并观察其动态反应。正常人,当眼受到光线刺激后瞳孔立即缩小,移开光源后瞳孔迅速复原。间接对光反射是指光线照射一侧瞳孔时,另一侧瞳孔立即缩小,移开光线,瞳孔扩大。

取手电筒,聚光后检查对光反射。手电光由外向内移动,直接照射左瞳孔,并观察瞳孔是否缩小。移开光源后,用手隔开双眼,再次用手电光直接照射左瞳孔并观察右侧瞳孔的动态反应。同法检查右侧。

瞳孔对光反射迟钝或消失,见于昏迷受检者。

Dilated pupils on both sides accompanied with disappearance of light reflection are signs of dying.

QR code 3-3　Pupillary light reflex

双侧瞳孔散大并伴有对光反射消失为濒死状态的表现。

二维码 3-3　瞳孔对光反射

3-4　Convergence Reflex

The examiner asks the examinee to look at his/her index finger from 1 m away, then gradually moves the index finger close to the bridge of the nose to about 5-10 cm away from the eyeballs. Normally, the two eyeballs are cohesive and the pupils are shrinking, which is called convergence reflex. When the oculomotor nerve function is damaged or the ciliary and medial rectus muscles are paralyzed, the convergence reflex may disappear。

QR code 3-4　Convergence reflex

3-4　集合反射

评估者嘱受检者注视1 m以外的食指,然后将食指逐渐向受检者鼻梁方向移动至距眼球5～10 cm处,正常人此时可见两眼球内聚,瞳孔缩小,称为集合反射。当动眼神经功能损害,睫状肌和双眼内直肌麻痹时,集合反射消失。

二维码 3-4　集合反射

Words and Expressions

binocular　*adj.* 双眼的

coma　*n.* 昏迷

conjunctiva　*n.* 结膜

dilate　*v.* 扩大,(使)膨胀,扩张

fornix　*n.* 穹,穹隆

illuminate　*vt.* 照射,照明,照亮

nystagmus　*n.* 眼球震颤

pupil　*n.* 瞳孔

sclera　*n.* 巩膜

sluggish　*adj.* 缓慢的,迟缓的,懒洋洋的

Assessment Skill 4
Thyroid Assessment

评估技能 4
甲状腺评估

Thyroid is a butterfly-shaped organ located below the thyroid cartilage and anterior to the trachea, extending to either side. It is soft, smooth, and impalpable. Thyroid assessment is generally carried out from three aspects: inspection, palpation and auscultation.

Inspection: The examinee takes a sitting or supine position. Normal thyroid is not visible. Mild enlargement can be seen in some adolescent girls. The examiner observes the size and symmetry of the thyroid, then instructs the examinee to swallow. Thyroid moves with the swallowing movement. Extending the neck can improve the visualization of thyroid.

Palpation: It includes examination of the thyroid isthmus and lateral lobes. Note the

甲状腺位于甲状软骨下方,气管两侧,左右对称,像蝴蝶形,表面光滑、柔软,不易触及。甲状腺评估一般从视诊、触诊、听诊三方面进行。

视诊:受检者取坐位或仰卧位,头后仰,正常甲状腺不可见,有些青春期少女可见轻微甲状腺肿大。评估者观察甲状腺的大小和对称性,嘱受检者做吞咽动作,可见甲状腺随吞咽动作而移动。受检者伸长颈部可以提高甲状腺的可见性。

触诊:包括甲状腺峡部和甲状腺侧叶的检查,触

contour and texture of the thyroid. Two methods can be adopted. For the anterior approach, the examiner stands in front of the examinee. Firstly, palpate the isthmus of the thyroid with one thumb. Start palpation from the suprasternal notch and slowly move upward, then ask the examinee to swallow a sip of water to feel for the upward movement of the isthmus. To palpate the lateral lobes, push the trachea to the opposite side with one thumb pressing on one side of the thyroid cartilage, then use the other thumb to palpate the lateral lobe with the posterior edge of sternocleidomastoid muscle pushed forward by the index and middle fingers of the same hand. Ask the examinee to swallow if thyroid is palpated. Repeat the procedure for the other lobe by reversing the hand. For the posterior approach, the examiner stands at the back of the examinee. Firstly, palpate the isthmus of the thyroid with the index finger. Start palpation from the suprasternal notch and slowly move upward, then ask the examinee to swallow a sip of water to feel for the upward movement of the isthmus. To palpate the lateral lobes, push the trachea with index and middle finger, and use the thumb of the other hand to squeeze the thyroid from the posterior edge of sternocleidomastoid muscle, the index finger and middle finger of the same hand to palpate the lateral lobe of thyroid. Ask the examinee to swallow if thyroid is palpated. Then

诊时注意甲状腺的轮廓和质地，一般采用双手触诊法检查甲状腺，双手触诊法又分前面触诊法和后面触诊法。前面触诊法：评估者站于受检者前面，用拇指从胸骨上切迹向上触摸甲状腺峡部，同时嘱受检者吞咽，感受峡部的上移，然后一手拇指施压于一侧甲状软骨，将气管推向对侧，另一手示指、中指在对侧胸锁乳突肌后缘向前推挤甲状腺侧叶，同侧手的拇指在胸锁乳突肌前缘触诊，注意配合吞咽动作，同法检查对侧。后面触诊法：评估者站于受检者后面，一手示指自胸骨上切迹向上触摸甲状腺峡部，同时嘱受检者吞咽，感受峡部的上移，然后，一手示指、中指将气管推向对侧，另一手拇指在对侧胸锁乳突肌后缘向前推挤甲状腺，同侧手的示指、中指在胸锁乳突肌前缘触诊甲状腺，注意配合吞咽动作，同法检查对侧。

check the opposite lobe with the same method.

Auscultation：There is no vascular murmur in normal thyroid. Among examinees with hyperthyroidism，systolic or continuous "buzz" can be heard. When touching the enlarged thyroid，the examiner should place the stethoscope directly on the enlarged thyroid and pay attention to whether there is vascular murmur.

听诊:正常甲状腺无血管杂音,甲状腺功能亢进者,可闻及收缩期或连续性"嗡鸣"音,当触及肿大的甲状腺时,用听诊器直接置于肿大的甲状腺上,注意有无血管杂音。

QR code 4　Thyroid assessment

二维码 4　甲状腺评估

Words and Expressions

cartilage　　*n.*软骨

contour　　*n.* 轮廓

hyperthyroidism　　*n.*甲状腺功能亢进

isthmus　　*n.* 地峡,峡部

sternocleidomastoid muscle　　胸锁乳突肌

suprasternal notch　　胸骨上切迹

texture　　*n.* 质地

thyroid　　*n.* 甲状腺

Assessment Skill 5
Thoracic and Pulmonary Assessment

评估技能 5
胸廓与肺脏评估

The purpose of chest assessment is to determine whether the thoracic organs are in physiological or pathological state. The examination of chest wall，thorax and breast is mainly performed by inspection and palpation，while the lungs should be examined in the sequence of inspection， palpation， percussion and auscultation.

胸部评估的目的是确定胸腔脏器有无病变，胸壁、胸腔和乳房的评估主要通过视诊和触诊进行，而肺脏的评估需要通过视诊、触诊、叩诊和听诊进行。

5-1 Thoracic Palpation

5-1-1 Thoracic Expansion

5-1-1-1 Anterior thoracic expansion：Thoracic expansion is to examine the movement range of the thorax during respiration. When checking the expansion of the anterior lower chest，place both hands on the chest with the extended thumbs lying along the inferior edges of the costal margins

5-1 胸廓触诊

5-1-1 胸廓扩张度

5-1-1-1 前胸胸廓扩张度：胸廓扩张度指呼吸时的胸廓活动度。检查前胸廓扩张度时，评估者双手置于受检者胸廓前下部对称位置，左右两拇指分别沿两侧肋缘指向剑突，手掌和其

pointing to xiphoid. The palms and the other fingers extend to the anterior chest wall. Ask the examinee to breathe deeply，watch the divergence of hands and feel the range and symmetry of respiratory movement.

余四指伸展置于前侧胸壁，嘱受检者做深呼吸，比较双手动度是否一致。

QR code 5-1-1-1　Anterior thoracic expansion

二维码 5-1-1-1　前胸廓扩张度

5-1-1-2　Posterior thoracic expansion：The examinee takes a sitting position with his/her back exposed. When checking the expansion of the posterior lower chest，place both thumbs at the level of the tenth rib and the thumbs should be parallel with vertebral spines. Pull hands medially until the thumbs meet over the vertebral spines. Ask the examinee to breathe deeply，watch the divergence of hands and feel the range and symmetry of respiratory movement.

5-1-1-2　后背胸廓扩张度：受检者取坐位，暴露背部。检查其背部胸廓扩张度时，双手平置于受检者背部，约第 10 肋骨水平，拇指与中线平行，将两侧皮肤推向中线，使拇指在中线汇合。嘱受检者做深呼吸，比较双手的动度是否一致。

QR code 5-1-1-2　Posterior thoracic expansion

二维码 5-1-1-2　后背胸廓扩张度

5-1-2　Chest Wall Palpation

Normally，there is no tenderness on the chest wall. Local tenderness of chest wall is usually found in intercostal neuritis，

5-1-2　胸壁触诊

正常人胸壁无压痛。胸壁局部压痛见于肋间神经炎、皮肌炎、肋软骨炎、外

dermatomyositis，costal chondritis，trauma and fracture. Sternal tenderness and percussion pain are common in leukemia examinees.

Pneumoderma is the air escaping and accumulating in the subcutaneous tissue of chest wall after the rupture of trachea，lung or pleura. The chest wall is swollen according to inspection. The movement of gas in the subcutaneous tissue can be felt by palpation and can result in crepitus or the feeling of holding snow.

5-1-3　Vocal Fremitus

5-1-3-1　Anterior vocal fremitus：Vocal fremitus is also perceived as vibratory palpation. During speech，the examinee's vocal cords sets up vibrations in the bronchial air column，which are conducted to the thoracic wall through lung septum and can be touched with hands. The examinee lies supine with the anterior chest exposed. The examiner puts fingers together and makes a light fist. Place the ulnar sides of the hands on the examinee's chest wall symmetrically and ask the examinee to repeat "yi". Touch the chest from top to bottom and avoid the heart from the third intercostal space. Feel the vibrations and compare symmetrical parts of the anterior chest from up to down. Pay attention to see if vocal fremitus is decreased or increased.

伤和骨折等。胸骨压痛和叩击痛见于白血病患者。

皮下气肿是指气管、肺或胸膜破裂后，气体逸出，积存于胸壁皮下组织。视诊见胸壁肿胀，触诊能感觉到气体在皮下组织移动，而出现捻发音或握雪感。

5-1-3　语音震颤

5-1-3-1　前胸语音震颤：语音震颤又称为触觉震颤，指受检者发出声音时，声波沿气管、支气管及肺泡传到胸壁引起的共鸣震动，可用手触及。受检者取仰卧位，暴露前胸部。评估者手指并拢轻握拳，双手掌尺侧缘轻放在受检者胸壁的对称部位，嘱受检者重复发"咿"的长音，从上到下触及前胸，于第 3 肋间开始注意避开心脏，比较两侧相应部位语音震颤是否对称，有无增强或减弱。

QR code 5-1-3-1　Anterior vocal fremitus

5-1-3-2　Lateral vocal fremitus：The examinee lies supine and puts arms up, exposing the lateral chest. The examiner puts fingers together and makes a light fist. Start below the armpit，place the ulnar sides of the hands on the examinee's lateral chest wall symmetrically and ask the examinee to repeat "yi". Touch the lateral chest from up to down. Feel the vibrations and compare symmetrical parts of the lateral chest. Pay attention to see if vocal fremitus is decreased or increased.

QR code 5-1-3-2　Lateral vocal fremitus

5-1-3-3　Posterior vocal fremitus：The examinee takes a sitting position with his/her back exposed， crossing hands over his/her shoulders. The examiner puts fingers together and makes a light fist. The examiner places the ulnar sides of the hands on the examinee's chest wall symmetrically and asks the examinee to repeat "yi". When palpating the interscapular area, place the ulnar edge of both hands between the scapula

二维码 5-1-3-1　前胸语音震颤

5-1-3-2　侧胸语音震颤：受检者仰卧位，双上臂上举，暴露胸部。评估者手指并拢轻握拳，从腋窝下方开始，双手尺侧缘轻放在受检者侧胸的对称部位，嘱受检者重复发"咿"的长音，从上到下，比较两侧相应部位语音震颤是否对称，有无增强或减弱。

二维码 5-1-3-2　侧胸语音震颤

5-1-3-3　后背语音震颤：受检者坐位，暴露背部。评估者手指并拢轻握拳，双手尺侧缘轻放在受检者背部的对称部位，自第一胸椎水平开始向下触诊，注意左右对称部位的比较，触诊肩胛间区时，双手尺侧缘置于肩胛骨和脊柱之间，嘱受检

and spine. Move the hands down to the lower edge of the thorax. Feel the vibrations and compare symmetrical parts of the back chest from up to down. Pay attention to see if there is a decrease or increase of vocal fremitus.

者重复发"咿"的长音,直至肩胛下角下方,从上到下触及背部,比较两侧相应部位语音震颤是否对称,有无增强或减弱。

QR code 5-1-3-3　Posterior vocal fremitus

二维码 5-1-3-3　后背语音震颤

5-1-4　Pleural Friction Fremitus

The examinee takes a supine or sitting position with chest exposed. The examiner puts fingers and palm together on the examinee's anterior inferior chest wall and ask him/her to take a deep breath. The pleural friction fremitus sounds like rubbing two pieces of leather together.

5-1-4　胸膜摩擦感

受检者仰卧位或坐位,暴露胸部。评估者手指并拢,双手分别置于受检者前下胸壁,嘱患者深呼吸,若双手有两层皮革相互摩擦的感觉即为有胸膜摩擦感。

QR code 5-1-4　Pleural friction fremitus

二维码 5-1-4　胸膜摩擦感

5-2　Pulmonary Percussion

Assist the examinee to relax and breathe calmly in a sitting or supine position. When percussing the anterior chest wall, the examinee should protrude forward his/her chest. When percussing the lateral chest wall, the examinee

5-2　肺脏叩诊

受检者平静呼吸,取坐位或仰卧位。检查前胸壁时,胸部稍向前挺;检查侧胸壁时,双臂抱头;检查背部时,上身略前倾,头稍低,

should hold his/her head with both arms. When percussing the back, the examinee should slightly lean forward while touching his/her elbows with crossed arms. Adopt the method of indirect percussion (mediate percussion). The pleximeter finger should be placed in the intercostal space and moved in the direction parallel to the ribs. However, the direction should be parallel to the spine when percussing the interscapular region. Percuss the chest symmetrically from top to down and from outside to inside. Firstly, percuss the anterior chest, then lateral chest, then the back. Compare the superior part with the inferior part and compare the left with the right.

5-2-1　Anterior Chest Wall Percussion

Assist the examinee to supine position, find the sternal angle first, then locate the first intercostal space. Start percussing from the first intercostal space of the left, then the first intercostal space of the right, then the second intercostal space of the right, the second intercostal space of the left, and so on, with the pleximeter finger moving like the Chinese character '弓'. From the third intercostal space, the heart area should be avoided.

双手交叉抱肘。采用间接叩诊法,板指应置于肋间隙处,沿肋骨平行的方向移动,而在肩胛间区叩诊时则移动方向应平行于脊柱,遵循自上而下、由外向内的顺序,依次叩诊前胸、侧胸和背部。注意上下、左右对照。

5-2-1　前胸叩诊

受检者取仰卧位,检查者先找到受检者胸骨角,继而找到第1肋间隙,自左侧第1肋间开始,向下逐个肋间叩诊,板指呈"弓"字形移动,注意左右对比。从第3肋间开始注意避开心脏。

QR code 5-2-1　Anterior chest wall percussion

二维码 5-2-1　前胸叩诊

5-2-2　Lateral Chest Wall Percussion

Assist the examinee to supine position, put both of his/her arms upward beside the head. Percuss from the left axilla intercostal space, move the pleximeter finger downward to the next intercostal space like the Chinese character '弓', compare the sound of the left with that of the right.

QR code 5-2-2　Lateral chest wall percussion

5-2-3　Posterior Chest Wall Percussion

Assist the examinee to sit and hold the shoulders with crossed arms, keep the head low. Firstly, find the seventh cervical vertebra, then find the first thoracic vertebra. Percuss from the left of the first thoracic vertebra with pleximeter finger parallel to the spine and move like Chinese character '弓', Compare the sounds on both sides. From the subscapular angle, the pleximeter finger should be put in the intercostal space, parallel to the intercostal space and moved in '弓' shape, compare the sounds on both sides.

5-2-2　侧胸叩诊

受检者取仰卧位，双臂上举，从左侧腋窝肋间隙开始，逐一于肋间"弓"字形移动板指向下一肋间进行叩诊，注意左右对比。

二维码 5-2-2　侧胸叩诊

5-2-3　背部叩诊

受检者取坐位，双手交叉抱肩低头，定位第 7 颈椎继而向下定位第一胸椎，从第 1 胸椎旁脊柱左侧开始向下叩诊，"弓"字形移动板指，板指应平行于脊柱，注意左右对比。叩诊至肩胛下角处，板指应放置于肋间隙处，平行于肋间走行，"弓"字形移动板指，注意左右对比。

QR code 5-2-3　Posterior chest wall percussion

二维码 5-2-3　背部叩诊

5-2-4　Inferior Boundary of Lung (along the right mid-clavicular line)

Assist the examinee to take a supine position and find the right mid-clavicular line. Percuss from the resonance area and move downward. keep on percussing downward, when the sound changing from resonance to dullness, it indicates that the upper boundary of liver has arrived. When the dullness changing to flatness, it indicates that the inferior lung boundary has arrived. Normally, the inferior margins of the lungs extend to the sixth interspace at the mid-clavicular line.

5-2-4　右锁骨中线肺下界叩诊

受检者取仰卧位,沿右锁骨中线由清音区逐一沿肋间向下叩诊,由清音变为浊音提示到达肝上界,继续向下叩诊,由浊音变实音到达肺下界。右锁骨中线上的肺下界一般在第6肋间。

QR code 5-2-4　Inferior boundary of lung
(along the right mid-clavicular line)

二维码 5-2-4　右锁骨中线
肺下界叩诊

5-2-5　Movement Range of the Inferior Lung Boundary (along the scapular line)

Assist the examinee to take a sitting position and hold the shoulders with crossed arms and keep the head low. Firstly, determine the level of

5-2-5　肩胛线肺下界移动度叩诊

患者取坐位,双手交叉抱肩,头下垂,评估者于其平静呼吸时在左侧肩胛线

the inferior lung boundary along the left scapular line during quiet respiration. Secondly，ask the examinee to take a deep breath and hold it，percuss downward until dullness replaces resonance and mark the level. Thirdly，ask the examinee to breathe calmly for a while and then exhale deeply and hold breath，percuss the inferior lung boundary again and mark the level. The distance between the two marks is the movement range of the inferior lung boundary. It is normally 6-8 cm. Then examine on the right side and compare with that of the left.

上叩出肺下界的位置（清音变为浊音），然后嘱患者深吸气后屏住呼吸，再次叩出肺下界，并做标记，然后嘱患者平静呼吸一会儿，之后深呼气，屏住呼吸，重新叩出肺下界并做标记。量出最高点与最低点之间的距离，此距离即为肺下界移动范围，正常为 6～8 cm。同法检查右侧。

QR code 5-2-5　Movement range of the inferior lung boundary（along the scapular line）

二维码 5-2-5　肩胛线肺下界移动度叩诊

5-3　Pulmonary Auscultation

Auscultation of the lungs comprises anterior chest，lateral chest and posterior chest auscultation.

5-3-1　Auscultation of Anterior Chest

Auscultate the lungs with the examinee in a sitting or supine position. It would be better to ask the examinee to fully expose the chest. Instruct the examinee to breathe more forcefully than usual. Use the stethoscope to auscultate the anterior chest. Begin at the left

5-3　肺脏听诊

胸部肺脏听诊主要包括前胸部听诊、侧胸部听诊和背部听诊。

5-3-1　前胸听诊

嘱受检者取坐位或仰卧位，完全暴露胸部。首先指导受检者做深呼吸，使用听诊器听诊受检者胸部肺脏的各个部分，自上而下，从前胸左侧第 1 肋间开始，

of the first intercostal space and move the chestpiece downward like the Chinese character '弓', auscultate in each intercostal space. Avoid the heart area from the third intercostal space. Compare symmetrical points sequentially，each part should be auscultated for at least one to two completed breathing cycles. During auscultation，pay attention to whether there is abnormal breath sounds，rales or pleural friction sounds. If exists，pay attention to its position, loudness and relationship with respiratory phases.

向下逐一肋间进行，"弓"字形移动听诊器体件，进行至第3肋间时应注意避开心脏，注意左右对称部位的比较。每个部位听诊至少1～2个完整的呼吸周期。听诊时，注意有无异常呼吸音、啰音或胸膜摩擦音，若有，注意其位置、大小以及与呼吸周期的关系。

QR code 5-3-1　Auscultation of anterior chest

二维码 5-3-1　前胸听诊

5-3-2　Auscultation of Lateral Chest

When auscultating the lateral chest, assist the examinee to take a supine position and ask the examinee to put both arms up, exposing lateral chest. The auscultation order of lateral chest is from armpit to costal margin at axillary midline. During auscultation, pay attention to the comparison of left and right symmetrical parts. Pay attention to whether there is abnormal breathing sounds，rales or pleural friction sounds. If exists，pay attention to its position，loudness and relationship with respiratory phases.

5-3-2　侧胸听诊

听诊侧胸时，患者取仰卧位，双上臂上举，侧胸的听诊顺序为自腋中线上腋窝开始，逐一沿肋间向下听诊，直至肋缘。听诊时，注意左右对称部位的对比，注意有无异常呼吸音、啰音或胸膜摩擦音，若有，注意其位置、大小以及与呼吸周期的关系。

QR code 5-3-2　Auscultation of lateral chest

二维码 5-3-2　侧胸听诊

5-3-3　Auscultation of Posterior Chest

To auscultate the back, assist the examinee to take a sitting position, holding his/her shoulder with crossed arms and keeping the head low. Find the seventh cervical vertebra, then the first thoracic vertebra. Auscultate from the left of the first thoracic vertebra and move the chestpiece like Chinese character '弓', compare the sounds on both sides. From the subscapular angle, the chestpiece should be put in the intercostal space and move in '弓' shape, compare the sounds on both sides. During auscultation, pay attention to whether there is an abnormal breathing sounds, rales or pleural friction sounds. If exists, pay attention to its position, loudness and relationship with respiratory phases.

5-3-3　背部听诊

背部听诊时,患者取坐位,双手交叉抱肩低头,评估者定位第 7 颈椎继而向下定位第一胸椎,从第一胸椎旁脊柱左侧开始向下听诊,"弓"字形移动听诊器,注意左右对比。听诊至肩胛下角处时,听诊器应放置于肋间隙处,"弓"字形移动听诊器体件,注意左右对比。听诊时,注意有无异常呼吸音、啰音或胸膜摩擦音,若有,注意其位置、大小以及与呼吸周期的关系。

QR code 5-3-3　Auscultation of posterior chest

二维码 5-3-3　背部听诊

Words and Expressions

armpit　　*n.*腋窝

axillary midline　　腋中线

cervical vertebra　　颈椎

clavicular　　*n.*锁骨的

costal margins　　肋缘

dermatomyositis　　*n.* 皮肌炎

divergence　　*n.*（意见、态度等的）分歧、差异

interscapular　　*adj.*肩胛间的

intercostal neuritis　　肋间神经炎

intercostal space　　肋间隙

leukemia　　*n.* 白血病

pleura　　*n.*胸膜

pleural friction sounds　　胸膜摩擦音

pneumoderma　　*n.* 皮下气肿

protrude　　v.突出,伸出,鼓出

rales　　*n.*啰音

scapula　　*n.*肩胛（骨）

scapular　　*adj.*肩胛的

septum　　*n.*隔膜

thoracic　　*adj.* 胸的,胸腔的,胸廓的

thorax　　*n.* 胸,胸廓,胸部

trachea　　*n.* 气管

sternal　　*n.* 胸骨

sternal angle　　胸骨角

subcutaneous　　*adj.* 皮下的

vertebra　　*n.*椎骨,脊椎

vocal fremitus　　语音震颤

Assessment Skill 6
Cardiac Assessment

评估技能 6
心脏评估

Heart assessment consists of four procedures：inspection，palpation，percussion and auscultation. The function of inspection is to determine the position and scope of apex impulse，while palpation further helps to determine the intensity of it. Through palpating，the presence of fremitus can be found. Percussion is mainly adopted to help determine the heart borders. Auscultation is the most important step in heart assessment. Through auscultation in each auscultatory area，we can detect the intensity of heart sound，the existence of arrhythmia or murmur.

心脏评估步骤分为视、触、叩、听。视诊侧重确定心尖搏动的位置和范围，触诊则进一步帮助确定心尖搏动的强度，还可判断心尖部有没有震颤。叩诊用于确定心界的大小。听诊是心脏查体最重要的步骤，各个瓣膜听诊区的听诊有助于判断心音的强度、有无心律失常或杂音。

6-1 Cardiac Inspection

6-1 心脏视诊

Cardiac inspection begins with the examinee in supine position. Sitting position is also acceptable for the examinee in the

心前区视诊可以取仰卧位或坐位，检查者站在受检者右侧，受检者充分暴露

outpatient. Examiner stands at the right side of the examinee with his/her chest fully exposed. Normal precordium area and the opposite should be symmetrical and without protrusion or excavation.

The apical impulse is formed by the apex regional vibration with the left ventricular systole. Normal apex impulse can be seen in the fifth left intercostal space at the tangent position，about 0.5-1.0 cm inside in the midclavicular line. The range of the impulse should be around 2.0-2.5 cm. In some special conditions，apical impulse is not seen. The scope and location of apex impulse could vary by examinee's body shape and position.

胸部。正常人心前区与右侧相应部位基本对称，无隆起或下陷。

心尖搏动是随着左心室的收缩而产生的心尖局部震动。受检者暴露心前区，检查者于切线位置观察其心尖搏动的位置及范围。正常人心尖搏动位于左侧第 5 肋间锁骨中线内侧 0.5～1.0 cm，其搏动范围的直径为 2～2.5 cm。少数正常人心尖搏动观察不到，人体位置及体型等的变化可使心尖搏动的范围及位置发生一定的生理变化。

QR code 6-1　Cardiac Inspection

二维码 6-1　心脏视诊

6-2　Cardiac Palpation

6-2-1　Palpation of Apical Impulse

Palpation can not only further determine the location，intensity and size of the apical impulse and abnormal precordial pulsations，but also reveal cardiac rate and rhythm.

6-2　心脏触诊

6-2-1　心尖搏动触诊

触诊不仅能进一步确定心尖搏动和心前区异常搏动的位置、强度和大小，而且可以确定心率和心律。

The examinee is in a supine position with the precordium area exposed. Examiner could apply his/her whole right palm to perform cardiac palpation. Using the pulp of index finger together with that of middle finger to determine the location where the impulse is the most obvious. The intensity，rate and rhythm of apical beat should be concerned. In some special conditions，apical impulse is impalpable when the examinee is obese，with mastoptosis and so on.

受检者取仰卧位,暴露心前区。评估者以右手手掌置于受检者心前区进行触诊,示指和中指并拢,以指腹确定心尖搏动最强点的位置、搏动范围,并注意心尖搏动的强弱、速率及节律。在一些特殊情况下,如肥胖、乳房下垂等,可触不到心尖搏动。

QR code 6-2-1　Palpation of apical impulse

二维码 6-2-1　心尖搏动触诊

6-2-2　Palpation of Thrill

Thrill is a sign of valve stenosis and some congenital heart diseases. The occurrence of vibration is due to the turbulence caused by the blood flowing through the narrow caliber or along the abnormal direction，which makes the vibration of valve，vascular wall or cardiac cavity wall transmitted to the chest wall. The intensity of the thrill depends on the velocity of the blood flow，the degree of narrowing of the orifice and the difference in pressure between the two chambers of the heart. It is also associated with chest wall thickness，the thinner the chest wall is，the easier to be palpated.

6-2-2　震颤触诊

震颤为瓣膜狭窄及某些先天性心脏病的特征性体征,血液经狭窄的口径或循异常的方向流动,形成旋涡,造成瓣膜、血管或心壁震动,传至胸壁产生震颤。震颤的强度与血流速度、瓣膜狭窄程度及心脏两腔室间压力差的大小有关,也与胸壁的厚薄有关,胸壁越薄,越容易触及震颤。

The examinee is in a supine position with the precordium area exposed. The examiner moves his/her palm against the precordium area. Remember not to press with force, as it could affect the sensitivity and result of palpation.

Thrill is hardly found in healthy individuals. Patients with kinds of heart disease could have thrill. Once detected, the examiner should pay attention to its location, time in cardiac cycle and mode of extension or transmission. The examiner can determine its time by palpating apical impulse or carotids impulse. Auscultation can also be applied to determine the relationship between thrill and heart sound.

受检者取仰卧位,暴露心前区,评估者将手掌紧贴心前区的不同部位进行触诊。切勿用力将手掌按压在胸壁上,因为用力按压可减低手上触觉感受器的敏感度,以至触不到震颤。

正常人心前区触不到震颤。心脏疾患患者可以触到震颤,若触及震颤,应注意其发生部位及时期(收缩期或舒张期),可以利用心尖搏动、颈动脉搏动、心音来帮助鉴别。

QR code 6-2-2　Palpation of thrill

二维码 6-2-2　震颤触诊

6-2-3　Pericardium Friction Rub

Pericardium friction rub doesn't exist in normal person and is caused by fibrinous pericarditis, in which visceral and parietal pericardium becomes coarse. It is easily palpated at the fourth left intercostal space. It usually can be palpated with the patient sitting erect or leaning forward during the end period of deep expiration.

6-2-3　心包摩擦感

正常人无心包摩擦感。当心包膜发生炎症时可产生心包摩擦感,一般在胸骨左缘第四肋间较易触及,前倾坐位时或深呼气后更易触及。

6-3　Percussion of Cardiac Dullness Border

Cardiac percussion can be adopted to confirm the heart borders，contour and its location in the thoracic cavity. The percussion on the bare area with no lungs tissue covered at the surface of the heart is flat，called as absolute cardiac dullness. The percussion on area covered by lungs tissue is dull，called as relative cardiac dullness. The real heart border is refer to relative cardiac dullness，which reflects the full size of heart.

The examinee is in a supine position with the thoracic part exposed. Indirect percussion is usually employed. Prepare two rulers，one soft ruler，two mark pens，one record card，and a pen. Draw the midline and the left midclavicularline first. The examiner uses his/her left middle finger as the pleximeter finger，parallels it to intercostal space when the examinee lies supine on an examining bed. During percussion，the examiner should press pleximeter finger firmly on the surface that is to be percussed，and percuss with the middle finger of right hand，then move medially until cardiac dullness is noticed.

Cardiac percussion starts from left to right，from outside to inside，and from the bottom up.

6-3　心脏浊音界叩诊

心脏相对浊音界的叩诊有助于确认心脏在胸腔的边界、轮廓和位置。心脏裸区即不被肺覆盖的区域，叩诊呈绝对浊音（实音）；其左右缘被肺覆盖的部分，叩诊呈相对浊音。叩诊心界指叩诊心脏相对浊音界，反映心脏的实际大小。

受检者取仰卧位，充分暴露胸部。叩诊方法为间接叩诊法。准备 2 把直尺、1 把软尺、2 支马克笔、1 份记录表和 1 支笔。用软尺画出前正中线和左锁骨中线。叩诊从左侧第 5 肋间心尖搏动外侧 2～3 cm处开始，叩诊板指与肋间平行。在叩诊过程中，检查者应将板指紧按在要叩诊部位，用右手中指叩诊，然后向内侧移动，直到出现浊音。

心脏叩诊的顺序为先左后右，从外向内，自下而上，逐一沿肋间进行叩诊，直到第 2 肋间。

Percussion of left border：It usually starts from 2-3 cm lateral to the point of maximal impulse，which is outlined by percussing in the 5th, 4th, 3rd, and the 2nd left intercostal space sequentially，starting from the anterior axillary line towards the sternum. Move the pleximeter finger less than 1 cm between each percussion. The point at which percussion note becomes dull represents the left heart border，and the beginner should mark with a mark pen where the note changes.

Percussion of right border：Percussion of upper margin of liver should be performed first along the right midclavicular line. Start from the second right intercostal space sequentially and move downward until liver dullness is noticed. The right heart border is outlined by percussing from one intercostal space above the upper margin of liver to the second right intercostal space sequentially，move medially until cardiac dullness is noticed. Mark the border with a mark pen.

At the end，the distance from mid-sternal line to the left and right border should be measured and recorded，the distance from mid-sternal line to left mid-clavicular line should also be measured，all data should be recorded as shown in table 6-1.

心脏左界的叩诊：一般从左侧第 5 肋间心尖搏动最强处外侧 2～3 cm 处开始，从腋前线向胸骨方向叩诊，由清音变为浊音处即为心脏边界，逐一沿肋间向上进行，直至第 2 肋间。叩诊板指移动距离每次不超过 1 cm。初学者要用笔做好标记。

心脏右界的叩诊：先叩出右锁骨中线上肝上界，在右锁骨中线第 2 肋间开始由上至下进行叩诊，清音变为浊音处为肝上界。由肝上界的上一个肋间开始，由外向内逐个肋间进行叩诊，标记由清音变浊音处，再依次逐个肋间上移，直至第二肋间为止。用马克笔进行标记。

叩诊完毕后用相互垂直的两把直尺测量出各肋间相对浊音界与前正中线的水平距离、左锁骨中线与前正中线的距离，并记录。将测量结果用表 6-1 所示的方式表示。

Table 6-1　The examinee's cardiac dullness border

Right heart border/cm	Intercostal space	Left heart border/cm
2	Ⅱ	3
2	Ⅲ	3.5
2.5	Ⅳ	5
—	Ⅴ	7.5

Note：The distance from mid-sternal line to left mid-clavicular line is about 8 cm.

表 6-1　受检者心脏相对浊音界

右心界/cm	肋间	左心界/cm
2	Ⅱ	3
2	Ⅲ	3.5
2.5	Ⅳ	5
—	Ⅴ	7.5

注:左锁骨中线距前正中线距离为 8 cm。

QR code 6-3　Percussion of cardiac dullness border

二维码 6-3　心脏浊音界叩诊

6-4　Cardiac Auscultation

Cardiac auscultation is one of the most important and difficult part of cardiac physical examination. Skilled cardiac auscultation is not only the basis for clinical diagnosis but also providing lots of information.

The examinee could take a sitting or

6-4　心脏听诊

心脏听诊是心脏体格检查最重要和最难的部分之一。评估者娴熟的心脏听诊技术不仅是临床诊断的基础,而且可以提供很多的信息。

患者可采取坐位、仰卧

supine position with full chest exposed during auscultation. If necessary, the examinee could change his/her position, hold the breath or implement appropriate physical activities to make some sounds or murmurs clearer. Prepare stethoscope, record card and pen.

Sounds produced by valve opening and closing may propagate to different areas. The clearest sound area is called auscultatory valve area, which is not equal to the valve anatomic location, which means that the auscultatory areas do not correspond with the surface markings of the heart valves. There are 5 auscultatory areas in cardiac auscultation, and their locations are as follows.

Mitral valve area (MV): Fifth intercostal space near the left midclavicular line, where the apex of the heart is located.

Aortic valve area (AV): Second intercostal space at the right sternal border.

The second aortic valve area: Third to fourth intercostal space at the left sternal border.

Pulmonic valve area (PV): Second intercostal space at the left sternal border.

Tricuspid valve area (TV): Fourth to fifth intercostal space at the left sternal border, which is also the left side of lower corpus of sternal.

Auscultatory valve area should be

位,必要时可变换体位、屏住呼吸或进行适当活动使得杂音更清晰。评估者准备听诊器、记录纸、笔。

瓣膜开合发出的声音可以传导至身体不同的部位,声音最响的部位为瓣膜听诊区,与瓣膜的解剖位置不一致,也就是说,听诊区与心脏瓣膜的体表标记位置不一致。有5个心脏瓣膜听诊区,它们的位置如下所示。

二尖瓣听诊区:多位于第5肋间左锁骨中线稍内侧,一般在心尖部。

主动脉瓣听诊区:胸骨右缘第2肋间。

主动脉瓣第二听诊区:胸骨左缘第3、4肋间。

肺动脉瓣听诊区:胸骨左缘第2肋间。

三尖瓣听诊区:胸骨左缘第4、5肋间,胸骨体下端左缘。

听诊瓣膜区可以根据

appropriately adjusted by the cardiac structure and position.

Cardiac auscultation should be started in a systematic way, usually in counter clockwise sequence: Starting from MV area, then PV area, then AV area, then second AV area, then TV area respectively. Firstly, auscultate the heart rate and rhythm in the mitral valve auscultation area for at least 1 minute, then auscultate each valve area in turn, and pay attention to the intensity and duration of the S_1 and the S_2. When auscultating the pulmonary valve auscultation area and aortic valve auscultation area, pay attention to the intensity comparision of P_2 and A_2, and note whether there is an additional heart sound and murmur. If murmur is heard, concern the location of the loudest murmur, occurrence cardiac period, nature, intensity, conduction, etc.

心脏的结构和位置的不同而发生改变。

听诊时,可按逆时针方向进行听诊,即二尖瓣区、肺动脉瓣区、主动脉瓣区、主动脉瓣第二听诊区、三尖瓣听诊区。首先在二尖瓣听诊区听诊心率、节律至少1分钟,再依次听诊各瓣膜区,注意第一心音(S_1)、第二心音(S_2)的强度、持续时间。在听诊肺动脉瓣听诊区和主动脉瓣听诊区时,应注意 P_2 与 A_2 强度的对比;同时,应注意有无额外心音及杂音。若闻及杂音,应注意杂音的最响部位、出现时期、性质、强度、有无传导等。

QR code 6-4　Cardiac auscultation

二维码 6-4　心脏听诊

Words and Expressions

aortic valve　主动脉瓣

apex　*n.* 心尖

arrhythmia　*n.* 无节律性,心律不齐(失常)

auscultatory　*adj.* 听诊的

border   *n.* 边界

caliber   *n.* 口径,量规,卡尺

carotids   *n.* 颈动脉

congenital   *adj.* 先天的,天生的

fibrinous pericarditis   纤维素性心包炎

intensity   *n.* 强度

mastoptosis   *n.* 乳房下垂

mitral valve   二尖瓣

pericardium friction rub   心包摩擦感

precordium   *n.* 心前,心前区,心窝

propagate   *v.* 宣传,传播,繁殖

pulmonic valve   肺动脉瓣

rhythm   *n.* 节律,规律,节奏

stenosis   *n.* 狭窄

supine position   仰卧位

tangent   *n.* 切线,正切

thrill   *n.* 震颤感 *v.* 使非常兴奋,使非常激动

tricuspid valve   三尖瓣

valve   *n.* 瓣膜,阀门,活塞

vortex   *n.* 旋涡

Assessment Skill 7
Abdomen Assessment

评估技能 7
腹部评估

Abdomen assessment is an important part of physical assessment. To avoid the impacts of palpations on the auscultation of bowel sounds, the sequence of abdomen assessment should be: inspection, auscultation, percussion and palpation.

腹部评估是身体评估重要的一部分。为了避免腹部触诊对于肠鸣音听诊的影响,腹部检查的顺序是视诊、听诊、叩诊、触诊。

7-1　Inspection

Before abdomen assessment, the examinee should empty the bladder. During inspection, the examinee takes a supine position, fully exposes the abdomen from the xiphoid process to the symphysis pubis. The examiner stands on the right side of the examinee and inspects the abdomen from top to bottom in a certain order. Abdomen inspection includes abdominal protuberance, respiratory movements, veins of abdominal wall, gastrointestinal pattern

7-1　腹部视诊

腹部视诊前,嘱受检者排空膀胱。视诊时,受检者取仰卧位,双手放于身体两侧,充分暴露全腹,暴露部位上自剑突,下至耻骨联合。评估者站在受检者的右侧,自上而下按照一定的顺序进行视诊。视诊的内容包括腹部外形、呼吸运动、腹壁静脉、胃肠型及蠕

and peristalsis, and states of abdominal wall, such as pigmentation, skin rash, abdominal striae, etc.

7-2 Auscultation

Abdomen auscultation includes auscultation of bowel sound, succession splash, and vascular murmur, etc.

7-2-1 Auscultation of Bowel Sound

The bowel sound is produced by gas and fluid flowing in the intestinal canal with intestinal peristalsis, which is a type of intermittent gurgling sound. Normal bowel sounds occur about 4-5 times per minute with a large difference among frequency, intensity, and pitch, most clearly heard in the umbilical region. Active bowel sounds, reaching up to over 10 times per minute and showing a relatively low pitch as peristalsis increases, are noted in acute gastroenteritis and after the administration of laxatives or in massive hemorrhage of gastrointestinal tract.

Explain to the examinee. Assist the examinee to take a supine position with knees bent and abdomen exposed. Prepare a stethoscope. Warm the stethoscope chestpiece with your hands first if it is cold. Listen to the bowel sound with stethoscope from the left lower quadrant in the counter clockwise direction. Finally focus on the umbilical region

动波,腹壁其他情况(如色素、皮疹、腹纹等)。

7-2 腹部听诊

腹部听诊包括肠鸣音、振水音和血管杂音等听诊。

7-2-1 肠鸣音听诊

肠蠕动时,肠管内的气体和液体随之流动,产生一种断续的咕噜声或气过水声,称为肠鸣音。正常肠鸣音每分钟有 4~5 次,以脐部最清楚。急性胃肠炎、服用泻药或胃肠道大出血时,会出现活跃的肠鸣音,每分钟达 10 次以上,随着蠕动的增加,肠鸣音的音调相对降低。

向受检者做好解释,受检者取屈膝仰卧位,暴露腹部。评估者准备好听诊器,如果环境温度较低,评估者可提前用手捂一下听诊器体件。用听诊器自左下腹开始以逆时针方向听诊腹部肠鸣音,最后将听诊器固

to auscultate bowel sound at least 1 minute. Pay attention to the frequency and intensity of the bowel sound. Pay attention to abnormal bowel sounds, such as active bowel sounds, hyperactive bowel sounds, hypoactive bowel sounds and absence of bowel sounds.

定在脐部,于脐部至少听诊1分钟。注意评估肠鸣音的次数和性质。评估有无肠鸣音异常的几种情况,如肠鸣音活跃、肠鸣音亢进、肠鸣音减弱和肠鸣音消失等。

QR code 7-2-1　Auscultation of bowel sound

二维码 7-2-1　肠鸣音听诊

7-2-2　Auscultation of Succession Splash

The examinee takes supine position with knees bent, while the examiner either puts one ear close to the examinee's upper abdomen or places the chestpiece of stethoscope here. Then the examiner impacts the examinee's upper abdomen fast and continuously with slightly curved fingers of right hand, which is called percussive palpation. If the examiner could hear the "clang" sound caused by the colliding of gas and fluid in the stomach, it is called succession splash.

7-2-2　振水音听诊

受检者取屈膝仰卧位,评估者一耳凑近受检者上腹部或将听诊器体件放于此处,然后用稍弯曲的手指以冲击触诊法连续迅速冲击受检者上腹部,胃内液体与气体相撞击的"咣啷"声,称为振水音。

QR code 7-2-2　Auscultation of succession splash

二维码 7-2-2　振水音听诊

7-2-3　Auscultation of Vascular Murmur

Normally, there is no vascular murmurs in the abdomen. Murmurs from arteries are often heard in the middle or one side of the abdomen. Aortic systolic murmur in the middle of the abdomen usually suggests abdominal aneurysm or abdominal aortic constriction. In aneurysm, the pulsatory mass can be felt here. Systolic blood murmur in both sides of the upper abdomen, is a sign of renal artery stenosis and occurs in young patients undergoing hypertension, while the murmur in both sides of the lower abdomen indicates iliac artery stenosis. When hepatic artery or abdominal aorta is compressed by left liver cancer, a blowing murmur can also be heard in the site of the mass or a mild continuous murmur is heard in the tumor position. Murmurs from veins sounds like a continuous hum, without systolic and diastolic properties, frequently appearing in the peripheral umbilicus or the upper abdomen.

The examinee takes supine position with knees bent. The examiner auscultated the upper part of the umbilicus, the left and right upper parts of the umbilicus, the left and right lower parts of the umbilicus and the groin of the examinee with a stethoscope to determine whether there is vascular murmur (Figure 7-1).

7-2-3　血管杂音听诊

正常人腹部无血管杂音。动脉的杂音常在腹部的中部或一侧听到。在腹部中部的主动脉收缩期杂音通常提示腹部动脉瘤或腹主动脉缩窄。在动脉瘤中,此部位可以触到搏动性肿块。上腹部两侧的收缩期血液杂音是肾动脉狭窄的标志,发生在年轻高血压患者中,而下腹部两侧的杂音表示髂动脉狭窄。当左肝癌压迫肝动脉或腹主动脉时,肿块部位也可听到吹风样杂音,或在肿瘤部位可听到轻微的持续性杂音。静脉杂音听诊有连续的"嗡嗡"声,经常出现在脐周或上腹部。

受检者取屈膝仰卧位,评估者用听诊器听诊脐部上方、脐左右上方、脐左右下方和腹股沟,确定有没有血管杂音(图 7-1)。

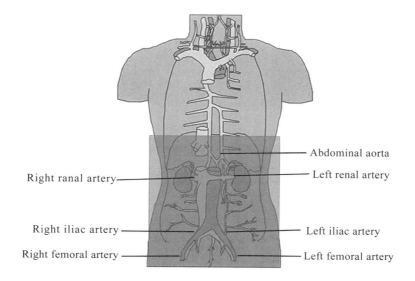

Figure 7-1　Auscultation locations of abdominal vessels

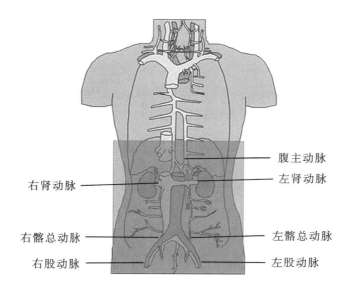

图 7-1　腹部血管杂音听诊部位

QR code 7-2-3　Auscultation of vascular murmur

二维码 7-2-3　血管杂音听诊

7-3　Percussion of the abdomen

Percussion of the abdomen is mainly to obtain the message of some disease such as abdomen tumors, inflation of the gastrointestinal tract, as well as the size of some organs, etc, usually cooperates with palpation to assist in judgement.

Percussion of abdomen can be performed by direct or indirect percussion, the latter is preferable for its better accurateness and reliability.

Percussion of abdomen includes abdominal percussion sound, upper and lower borders of the liver, percussion tenderness at hepatic region, percussion tenderness at costovertebral angle, bladder percussion and shifting dullness, which will be explained respectively.

7-3-1　Abdominal Percussion Sound

Percussion of abdomen is usually performed by indirect percussion. Normally, in the abdomen, the most common percussion sound is tympany. However, in the position of liver, spleen, enlarged bladder and uterus as well as in the abdominal flanks proximal to psoas,

7-3　腹部叩诊

腹部叩诊主要用于获取一些疾病的信息，如腹部肿瘤、胃肠道胀气以及一些腹部器官的大小等，通常配合触诊作为辅助判断。

腹部叩诊分为直接叩诊和间接叩诊，后者较常用，且准确性和可靠性更高。

腹部叩诊包括腹部叩诊音、肝上下界的叩诊、肝区叩击痛、肋脊角叩击痛、膀胱叩诊和移动性浊音的叩诊，以下分别对其进行讲述。

7-3-1　腹部叩诊音

采用间接叩诊法叩诊腹部。正常情况下，除肝脏、脾脏、增大的膀胱、子宫所占据的部位及两侧腹部近腰肌处为浊音或实音外，其余部位均为鼓音。

percussion sound is usually dullness or flatness.

Explain to the examinee. The examinee lies supine with knees bent, exposing the abdomen.

The abdominal percussion can be started from the left lower quadrant, and then to the right lower quadrant counterclockwise, finally in the umbilicus.

QR code 7-3-1　Abdominal percussion sounds

7-3-2　Upper and Lower Borders of the Liver

Explain to the examinee. The examinee lies supine with knees bent, exposing the throacoabdominal region and breathing calmly. To assess the upper border, percuss from the upper right chest along the right midclavicular line and percuss downward, noting the change from lung resonance to liver dullness. To assess the lower border, start percussing upward in the right lower quadrant along the mid-clavicular line. Continue percussing upward and note the change from tympany to dullness. Normally, along the right midclavicular line, the upper border lies at the 5th intercostal space and the lower at the right subcostal margin, the distance is called liver span, which is about 9-11 cm.

向受检者做好解释,受检者取屈膝仰卧位,双手置于身体两侧,暴露腹部。

一般从左下腹部开始,沿逆时针方向叩诊腹部一周,最后叩诊脐部。

二维码 7-3-1　腹部叩诊音

7-3-2　肝脏上下界叩诊

受检者取屈膝仰卧位,暴露胸腹部,平静呼吸。评估者沿右锁骨中线由肺清音区往下叩诊至出现浊音,即为肝上界。评估者再由腹部鼓音区沿右锁骨中线向上叩至浊音处,即为肝下界。在右锁骨中线上,正常人上界位于第 5 肋间,下界位于右肋缘,肝上界和肝下界之间的距离,为肝浊音区上下径。一般匀称体型者的肝浊音区上下径为 9～11 cm。

The lower hepatic boundary overlaps with the stomach and colon, which makes it difficult to percuss accurately. Thereby, it is often determined by palpation.

由于肝下界与胃、结肠等重叠,很难叩准确,故常采用触诊确定。

QR code 7-3-2　Percussion of upper and lower borders of the liver

二维码 7-3-2　肝脏上下界叩诊

7-3-3　Percussion Pain at Hepatic Region

The examinee takes supine position with knees bent, the examiner places the left hand flat on the hepatic region, then uses the ulnar side of the right fist to strike the left hand with light to medium force. Normally, there is no percussion pain at the hepatic region.

7-3-3　肝区叩击痛

受检者取屈膝仰卧位,评估者将左手掌平放于肝区,右手握拳,用轻到中等力量叩击左手背。正常人肝区无叩击痛。

QR code 7-3-3　Percussion pain at hepatic region

二维码 7-3-3　肝区叩击痛

7-3-4　Percussion Tenderness at Costovertebral Angle

The examinee takes a sitting or lateral position, the examiner places the left hand flat on the costovertebral angle, then uses the ulnar side of the right fist to strike the left hand with light to medium force. Normally, there is no

7-3-4　肋脊角叩击痛

受检者取坐位或侧卧位,评估者以左手掌平放于受检者肋脊角处(肾区),右手握拳,用轻到中等力量叩击左手背。正常人肋脊角

percussion pain at the costovertebral angle.

处无叩击痛。

QR code 7-3-4　Percussion tenderness at costovertebral angle

二维码 7-3-4　肋脊角叩击痛

7-3-5　Bladder Percussion

The examinee takes supine position with knees bent. Bladder percussion is used to determine the degree of urinary bladder distention，which is generally carried out above the pubic symphysis，with tympany shifting to dullness from the top down. Then percuss from the lateral to the bladder area. When the bladder is empty, the percussion sound is tympany above the pubic symphysis，while when the bladder is full of urine, the percussion sound is dullness, showing oval-shaped or round.

7-3-5　膀胱叩诊

受检者取屈膝仰卧位，暴露腹部。膀胱叩诊适用于确定膀胱扩张的程度，评估者自耻骨联合上方腹部鼓音区开始向下叩诊至浊音区，再从左右侧方叩向膀胱区。膀胱空虚时，耻骨联合上方叩诊呈鼓音；膀胱充盈时，耻骨联合上方叩诊呈椭圆形或圆形浊音区。

QR code 7-3-5　Bladder percussion

二维码 7-3-5　膀胱叩诊

7-3-6　Percussion of Shifting Dullness

Due to gravity, fluid in the abdominal cavity mostly accumulates in the lower part of the abdominal cavity and floats with the body position. When the examinee takes the supine

7-3-6　移动性浊音叩诊

腹腔内液体因重力关系多潴留于腹腔的低处，并随体位而移动。受检者取仰卧位时，腹部两侧呈浊

position，dullness appears on both sides of the abdomen. With lateral position, dullness appears at the lower abdomen. The phenomenon that the dullness changes due to different positions is called shifting dullness.

Firstly, the examinee should take supine position with knees bent. The examiner percusses at the umbilical level from mid abdomen to the right side of the examinee. Once tympany shifts to dullness, hold the pleximeter finger still，then ask the examinee to turn and lie on his left side. After a moment，percuss the same point again. If it is still dullness，no shifting dullness is proved. But if the sound changes from dullness to tympany，it implies that the dullness has been shifted to another position. The examiner continues to percuss toward the examinee's left side until the tympany changes to the dullness. Hold the pleximeter finger still，and ask the examinee to take supine position，wait a moment and then percuss the same point. If the sound changes from dullness to tympany，shifting dullness is proved.

音;取侧卧位时,下侧腹部转为浊音。因体位不同而出现的浊音区变动的现象,称为移动性浊音。

受检者取屈膝仰卧位,评估者自受检者脐开始叩诊,向受检者右侧移动,至由鼓音变为浊音时,固定板指,嘱受检者取左侧卧位,稍停片刻,重新叩诊该处,若仍为浊音,提示为阴性;若由浊音变为鼓音,向左侧继续叩诊,当叩诊音由鼓音变为浊音时,固定叩诊板指,嘱受检者平卧,稍停片刻,重新叩诊该处,若由浊音变为鼓音,即为移动性浊音阳性。

QR code 7-3-6　Percussion of shifting dullness

二维码 7-3-6　移动性浊音叩诊

7-4　Abdomen Palpation

As a major method of abdominal examination, palpation plays a very significant role in recognition of abdominal signs. The examinee takes supine position with both legs slightly separated and flexed so that abdominal muscles can be fully relaxed. Ask the examinee to calmly conduct abdominal breathing and expose the abdomen. The examiner stands on the right side of the examinee.

Abdomen palpation includes light and deep palpation, tenderness and rebound tenderness, palpation of liver, palpation of spleen, and palpation of gallbladder, etc.

7-4-1　Light and Deep Palpation of Abdomen

The examinee takes a supine position. The examiner stands on the right side of the examinee. The sequence of palpation generally starts from the left lower abdomen to all areas of the abdomen successively in a counterclockwise direction. Light palpation first, then deep palpation. Pay attention to the examinee's reactions and expressions when palpating. If the examinee has complained of pain, palpate the healthy side first.

Light palpation is usually used to detect the tenseness and resistance of the abdominal wall, superficial tenderness, lumps, pulsation

7-4　腹部触诊

作为腹部检查的主要方法,触诊在发现腹部异常体征方面起到非常重要的作用。受检者取屈膝仰卧位,双腿稍分开,以充分放松腹肌,让受检者行平静腹式呼吸,评估者站于受检者右侧。

腹部触诊通常包括浅触诊、深触诊、压痛、反跳痛、肝脏触诊、脾脏触诊和胆囊触诊等。

7-4-1　腹部浅触诊和深触诊

受检者取屈膝仰卧位,检查者站在受检者右侧。腹壁触诊一般由左下腹开始,呈逆时针方向,陆续触诊其他区域,首先进行浅触诊,然后进行深触诊。触诊中应注意观察受检者的反应和表情。如受检者在触诊前已出现腹部疼痛,则应先触诊其他的正常区域。

浅触诊一般用于触诊腹壁紧张度、抵抗感,浅表的压痛、包块、搏动和腹壁

and masses on the abdominal wall. Deep palpation is used to detect the size and shape of the organs，tenderness，rebound tenderness and the masses in the abdominal cavity.

When conducting light palpation，hold the fingers of the right hand straight and keep them together. Gently press the abdominal wall with the flat part or the finger pulp of the right hand. The abdominal wall should be pressed down to a depth of about 1 cm，while conducting deep palpation，the depth should be more than 2 cm. Normal abdominal wall is usually soft. When palpating，check whether the tenseness of the whole abdomen or local abdominal wall is increased or decreased.

QR code 7-4-1　Light and deep palpation of abdomen

7-4-2　Tenderness and Rebound Tenderness

The examinee takes supine position with both legs slightly separated and flexed so that abdominal muscles can be relaxed fully. Ask the examinee to calmly perform abdominal breathing and expose abdomen. The examiner stands on the right side of the examinee.

The examiner presses the abdomen slowly from light to deep，asks the examinee

上的肿块。深触诊一般用于触诊脏器的大小、形态、压痛、反跳痛及腹腔内的包块等。

浅触诊时，将右手手指并拢，用右手的平展部分或指腹轻轻按压腹壁，下压腹壁深度在1 cm左右。深触诊时下压腹壁深度达2 cm以上。正常人腹部柔软，检查时注意有无全腹或局部腹壁紧张度增加、减低。

二维码 7-4-1　腹部浅触诊和深触诊

7-4-2　腹部压痛及反跳痛

受检者取屈膝仰卧位，双腿稍分开，以充分放松腹肌。受检者取平静腹式呼吸，评估者站于受检者右侧。

评估者由浅入深触压腹部，注意受检者有无腹部

whether there is pain. If pain is confirmed, keep the fingers still on the painful point for a moment, then quickly lift the fingers. Ask the examinee whether the pain aggravates.

QR code 7-4-2 Tenderness and rebound tenderness

7-4-3 Liver Palpation

Both single hand palpation and bimanual palpation can be applied to palpate liver. Bimanual palpation will be discussed as an example.

The examinee takes supine position with knees bent, relax the abdominal wall and expose the abdomen, then adopts deep and uniform abdominal breathing to make the liver move up and down along with the movement of diaphragm. When palpating the liver, pay attention to its size, texture, edge, surface smoothness and tenderness.

The examiner stands on the right side of the examinee and holds the examinee's right waist with left hand and places the hand on the costal region with thumb open. On palpation, the examiner pushes the left hand upward in order to make the inferior border of liver adhere closely to anterior abdominal wall.

压痛,若有压痛,手指在有压痛的部位稍停片刻,使压痛感趋于稳定,然后将手指迅速抬起,检查受检者有无反跳痛。

二维码 7-4-2 腹部压痛及反跳痛

7-4-3 肝脏触诊

肝脏触诊可采用单手触诊法或双手触诊法。下面将以双手触诊法为例来进行讲解。

嘱受检者取屈膝仰卧位,放松腹壁,暴露腹部,做较深而均匀的腹式呼吸,使肝脏随膈肌运动而上下移动。触诊肝脏时,注意其大小、质地、边缘情况、表面光滑度和压痛等。

评估者站于受检者右侧,将左手手掌置于受检者右腰部,将肝脏向上托起,拇指置于右季肋部,右手平置于右锁骨中线上肝下缘的下方(一般从脐水平线开始),4 指并拢,掌指关节伸

The examiner puts the right hand on the right midclavicular line, with 4 fingers closing together, metacarpophalangeal joint straight and the index finger and the middle finger pointing to the costal margin or the front of the index finger's radial side parallel to the costal margin. Usually palpate from the umbilical level upward. Liver palpation should coordinate with the examinee's abdominal breathing movements. As the examinee exhales, the examiner presses down on the abdominal wall and deeply palpate the edge of liver; as the examinee inhales, the examiner slowly lifts the fingers and meanwhile palpates the liver edge which is moving toward the costal margin with the tips of fingers. Repeat until the liver edge or costal margin is palpated. Palpate the left lobe of liver on the anterior median line with the same method.

直,示指与中指的指端指向肋缘或示指前端的桡侧与肋缘平行,与受检者的呼吸运动紧密配合进行触诊。受检者深呼气时,指端随之压向深部;深吸气时,触诊的手随腹壁抬起,并以指端向前上迎触下移的肝脏。如此反复进行,自下而上逐渐触向肋缘,直到触及肝缘或肋缘为止。用同样的方法于前正中线上触诊肝左叶。

QR code 7-4-3　Liver palpation

二维码 7-4-3　肝脏触诊

7-4-4　Spleen Palpation

Normally, spleen is not palpable, if is, it manifests descent of the diaphragm, which could result from pneumothorax or pleural effusion on the left side, or downward displacement of internal organs. In those

7-4-4　脾脏触诊

正常情况下,触诊无法触及脾脏,当发生内脏下垂、左侧胸腔积液或积气等,导致膈肌下降时,脾脏可随之向下移位,在受检者

cases, the edge of spleen could be palpated at the costal margin at the end of deep inhaling. When the disease causes splenomegaly, the spleen can also be touched.

Both single hand palpation and bimanual palpation can be adopted to palpate spleen. We'll take bimanual palpation for example.

During the bimanual palpation, the examinee can take either supine position or right lateral position. When the examinee takes supine position with knees bent, the examiner stands at the examinee's right side, reaches over the abdomen with the left arm, and places the left hand palm on the 9-11 ribs below the left chest, exerting pressure to move the posterior aspect of the chest anteriorly in order to limit thoracic movement. Meanwhile, the examiner places his/her right palm flat on the umbilicus from which palpation starts and keeps it roughly vertical with the left costal arch, which is similar to the maneuver used to palpate the liver. With the cooperation of the examinee's respiration, the examiner gradually pushes the right hand upward to feel the spleen tip, till the left costal margin. When the examinee is in the right lateral position, ask the examinee to straighten the right leg and bend the knee and hip of the left leg. the examiner stands at the examinee's right side. The procedures are the same as those of the supine position.

深吸气时可在肋缘下触及脾脏边缘。疾病导致脾脏肿大的情况下,脾脏也可被触及。

可采用单手或双手触诊,下面将以双手触诊法为例来进行讲解。

受检者可以取仰卧位或右侧卧位两种体位。受检者取仰卧位时,评估者位于受检者右侧,左手绕过受检者腹前方,手掌置于其左胸下部第9~11肋处,将脾脏由后向前托起。右手掌平置于脐周,与肋弓大致呈垂直方向,如同肝脏触诊,配合呼吸,迎触脾脏,直至触及脾缘或左肋缘。受检者取右侧卧位时,嘱其伸直右下肢,左下肢屈膝屈髋。其余方法同仰卧位双手触诊法。

QR code 7-4-4   Spleen palpation

7-4-5   Gallbladder Palpation

Normally, the gallbladder cannot be palpated. Gallbladder enlargement should be noticed when palpating. Sometimes the inflamed gallbladder does not enlarge, or does enlarge but remains above the costal margin. In those cases above, the gallbladder cannot be palpated but tenderness could be detected.

To test for Murphy's sign, ask the examinee to take supine position with knees bent. The examiner places the left palm on the examinee's right lower chest with the thumb pulp hooked at the gallbladder point (at the junction of the right costal margin and the outer margin of the rectus abdominis) with moderate pressure, and then asks the examinee to inhale slowly and deeply. During inspiration, inflamed gallbladder that descends will impact the hard-pressing thumb. As a result, the examinee will feel pain or stop inhaling because of the pain. It is the indication of Murphy's sign positive.

二维码 7-4-4   脾脏触诊

7-4-5   胆囊触诊

正常情况下,胆囊不能被触及。触诊时应注意有无胆囊肿大,但是某些胆囊炎症受检者胆囊未肿大或虽肿大但未及肋弓下缘,不能触及胆囊,但此时可有触痛。

墨菲征的检查方法:受检者取屈膝仰卧位,评估者将左手掌平放在受检者的右前下胸部,拇指指腹以中等度压力勾压于右肋缘与腹直肌外缘交界处,然后嘱受检者缓慢深吸气。如果在吸气过程中,有炎症的胆囊下移时碰到用力按压的拇指,即可引起疼痛或因剧烈疼痛而中止吸气,即为墨菲征阳性。

QR code 7-4-5　Gallbladder of palpation
　　　　　　　　　　　　　　　　　　　　二维码 7-4-5　胆囊触诊

Words and Expressions

abdomen　*n*. 腹部

abdominal flanks　腹侧

aggravate　*v*. 使……严重,使……恶化,激怒

bladder　*n*. 膀胱

bowel　*n*. 肠,内部最深处

colon　*n*. 结肠

costovertebral angle　肋脊角

counterclockwise　*n*. 逆时针方向

diaphragm　*n*. 膈,膈膜,横膈膜

gallbladder　*n*. 胆囊

gastrointestinal　*adj*. 胃肠的

gastroenteritis　*n*. 胃肠炎

hemorrhage　*n*.（尤指大量的）出血,失血　*vi*. 大出血

hepatic region　肝区

hyperactive　*adj*. 过分活跃的,多动的

hypoactive　*adj*. 活动力减退的

intermittent gurgling sound　断断续续的咕噜声

intestinal　*adj*. 肠的

laxatives　*n*. 轻泻药

liver　*n*. 肝脏

lumps　*n*. 肿块,隆起　*v*. 把……归在一起

Murphy's sign　默菲征

peristalsis　*n*.（肠等的）蠕动

pigmentation　*n*. 色素沉着

pleural effusion　胸膜腔积液

pneumothorax　*n*. 气胸

protuberance　*n*. 突出物,隆起部分

proximal　*adj*. 近端的,近身体中心的

psoas　*n*. 腰大肌,腰肌

pubic symphysis　耻骨联合

pulsation　*n*. 搏动,脉冲,脉动

quadrant　*n*. 四分之一圆,象限

rash　*n*. 皮疹,疹

rectus abdominis　腹直肌

stomach　*n*. 胃

spleen　*n*. 脾脏

stria　*n*. 条纹,细沟,线纹

succession splash　振水音

umbilical　*adj*. 脐带的,中央的

umbilical region　脐部

umbilicus　*n*. 脐,肚脐

uterus　*n*. 子宫

waist　*n*. 腰部

xiphoid process　剑突

Assessment Skill 8
Assessment of Spine and Extremities

评估技能 8
脊柱四肢评估

Spine and extremities assessment includes the following items: the examination of the spine, limbs and joints. The commonly used physical examination techniques in this part are inspection, palpation and percussion. A professional percussion hammer is needed in the percussion.

脊柱四肢的检查包括脊柱、四肢和关节的评估,本部分常用的体格检查手法是视诊、触诊和叩诊,其中叩诊需要借助叩诊锤来完成。

8-1　Vertebral Column Assessment

8-1　脊柱检查

The examinee should be in a standing or sitting position, with both upper limbs hanging naturally and undressed to fully expose the vertebral column.

受检者可取站立位或坐位,双上肢自然下垂,脱去上衣以充分暴露脊柱。

8-1-1　Spinal Curvature

8-1-1　脊柱弯曲度

8-1-1-1　Inspection: The examiner observes the examinee from one side. Normally, people have four physiological curvatures of the spine (cervical lordosis, thoracic kyphosis, lumbar

8-1-1-1　视诊:评估者从侧面进行视诊,正常人脊柱有四个生理弯曲(颈椎前凸、胸椎后凸、腰椎前凸、骶

61

lordosis，and sacral kyphosis).

8-1-1-2　Palpation：The examiner presses along the spinous process with her/his right thumb from top to bottom. After that，the skin will appear one red hyperemia line. Observe whether the red line is curved.

8-1-2　Spinal Mobility

8-1-2-1　Cervical vertebra：Fix the shoulders of the examinee，and normal cervical vertebrae could autonomously perform forward flexion (35°-45°)，extension (35°-45°)，lateral flexion (45°)，and rotation (60°-80°).

8-1-2-2　Lumbar vertebra：Fix the hip of the examinee，and the normal lumbar vertebra could autonomously perform forward flexion (75°-90°)，extension（30°），lateral flexion (20°-35°)，and rotation (30°).

QR code 8-1-2　Spinal mobility

8-1-3　Spinal Tenderness

The examiner presses the spinous process, interspinous ligament，and paravertebral muscle of each spine from top to bottom with the right

椎后凸）。

8-1-1-2　触诊：评估者用右手拇指沿着脊椎的棘突用适当的压力自上而下划压，划压后皮肤出现一条红色的充血线，观察红线有无侧弯。

8-1-2　脊柱活动度

8-1-2-1　颈椎：受检者肩部固定，正常人颈椎可自主进行前屈（35°～45°）、后伸（35°～45°）、左右侧弯（45°）以及左右旋转（60°～80°）动作。

8-1-2-2　腰椎：受检者髋部固定，正常人腰椎可自主进行前屈（75°～90°）、后伸（30°）、左右侧弯（20°～35°）以及左右旋转（30°）动作。

二维码 8-1-2　脊柱活动度

8-1-3　脊柱压痛

评估者用右手拇指自上而下逐个按压每个脊柱的棘突、棘间韧带和椎旁肌

thumb and asks the examinee if there is tenderness. If tenderness is present，the position of the affected vertebra should be recorded.

8-1-4　Percussion Pain

8-1-4-1　Direct percussion：The examinee sits up and the examiner stands behind him/her. With the help of a percussion hammer，the examiner tapes the spinous process of thoracic vertebra and lumbar vertebra from top to bottom and asks if there is percussion pain. If percussion pain is present，the position of the affected vertebra should be recorded.

8-1-4-2　Indirect percussion：The examinee sits up and the examiner places the left palm on the top of the examinee's head，and taps on the back of the left hand with the right fist's hypothenar，checking if there is pain. Pain elicited by percussion may reveal spinal tuberculosis，fractures or disc herniation.

8-2　Assessment of Limbs and Joints

Inspection and palpation are often used to check the shape of limbs and joints，position of limbs，mobility or movement，etc.

8-2-1　Joints of Upper Limbs

Neck，shoulders，elbows，wrists and hands are closely linked in anatomy as well as physiology and pathology. These parts need to

肉,询问受检者有无压痛。如有压痛,则记录病变椎体的位置。

8-1-4　叩击痛

8-1-4-1　直接叩击法：嘱受检者坐正,评估者站其身后,借助叩诊锤自上而下逐个叩击胸椎和腰椎棘突,询问受检者有无叩击痛。如有叩击痛,则记录病变椎体的位置。

8-1-4-2　间接叩击法：嘱受检者坐正,评估者将左手掌置于受检者头顶,右手握拳叩击左手背,询问受检者有无疼痛,若有疼痛,则受检者可能有脊柱结核、骨折或椎间盘突出。

8-2　四肢和关节的评估

常用视诊和触诊检查四肢及关节的形态、肢体位置、活动度或运动等情况。

8-2-1　上肢关节

颈部、肩、肘、腕和手不仅在解剖结构上紧密联系,而且在生理和病理功能上

be considered as a whole.

8-2-1-1 Shoulders: When examining the shoulders, it is important to have the examinee remove enough clothing so that both shoulders can be viewed and compared completely. Observe any asymmetry and any evidence of movement restriction. Inspect the contour of sternoclavicular and acromioclavicular joints to search for any evidence of swelling or deformity.

The range of motion in the shoulders should be assessed both actively and passively. Adduction is measured by having the examinee touch the opposite ear with elbow close to anterior chest wall. Flexion, abduction and external rotation are measured by having the examinee's hand reach behind the head and touch the opposite ear. Conversely, internal rotation and adduction of the shoulder should be tested by having the examinee's hand touch the inferior aspect of the opposite scapula from the back.

Besides local lesions in the shoulder, pain in the shoulder may result from neck nerve root irritation due to compression or inflammation. Visceral disorders may also refer the pain to the shoulder, known as referred pain. There is no tenderness in the shoulder and no restriction of motion in these disorders.

也密不可分,应将这些部位作为一个整体来考虑。

8-2-1-1 肩关节:检查肩关节时,要让受检者脱去衣物以便于检查双侧并进行对比,观察是否对称和有无活动受限。检查胸锁关节和肩锁关节有无肿胀和变形。

评估肩部的主动和被动运动范围。内收的评估方法是让受检者用肘靠近前胸壁,接触对侧耳朵。屈曲、外展和外旋通过受检者的手伸到头部后面并触摸对面的耳朵进行评估。相反,应通过让受检者的手从背部接触对侧肩胛骨的下侧评估肩部的内旋和内收。

除了肩部的局部损伤外,肩部疼痛可能是由压迫或炎症引起的颈部神经根刺激所致。内脏疾病也可能放射至肩部疼痛,称为放射痛。在这些疾病中,肩部没有压痛,运动也不受限制。

8-2-1-2　Elbows：When examining the elbows，it is important to compare both sides. Compare the size of the elbows，looking for asymmetry，etc.

When the elbow joint is extended，the tip of the olecranon and the humeral epicondyles should lie on a straight line. When the elbow is flexed，the olecranon descends until its tip forms the apex of an approximately equilateral triangle，of which the epicondyles form the angles at its base. These normal relationships are dismissed in dislocation of the elbow joint and arthritis. However，these relationships will not change in case of humeral fracture.

8-2-1-3　Wrists and Hands

Wrists：Compare both sides and look for deficits in the range of motion. Wrist motion can reach dorsal extension for 35°-60° and palmar flexion for 50°-60° without causing pain. Ask the examinee to hold their wrists in complete flexion by pushing the dorsal surfaces of both hands together，then in complete extension by pushing the palm of both hands together. Limitation of any motion is a feature of wrist arthritis，wrist fracture or dislocation.

Hands：Hands are vulnerable to mild injury. The skin of the palm is thick and connected to the skeleton by a layer of fibrous

8-2-1-2　肘关节：当评估肘关节时，进行双侧对比很重要，要比较双侧肘关节的大小、是否对称等。

当肘关节伸展时，鹰嘴尖端和肱骨上髁应位于一条直线上。当肘部弯曲时，鹰嘴下降，直到其尖端形成近似等边三角形的顶点，其中上髁形成其底部的角度。这些位置关系在肘关节脱位和关节炎中会消失。然而，在肱骨骨折的情况下，这些关系不会改变。

8-2-1-3　腕关节和手

腕关节：注意双侧比较，评估有无活动范围受限。手腕背伸可达到35°～60°，掌屈可达50°～60°，而不会引起疼痛。要求受检者通过将双手的背面合在一起来保持手腕完全弯曲，然后通过将双手的手掌合在一起来保持手腕完全伸展。任何运动受限都是腕关节炎、腕关节骨折或脱位的表现。

手：手容易受到伤害。手掌的皮肤很厚，通过一层纤维结缔组织（筋膜）与骨

connective tissue（fascia），while the skin of the dorsum is thin and movable so that fingers can flex. The lymphatic tissue is located in the dorsum of the hand. That is why the dorsum swells more significantly than the palm in case of hand inflammation.

Functional position of the hand is that wrist is in 30° dorsiflexion and 15° ulnar deviation，the thumb is abducted and opposite to the pads of the fingers，the proximal interphalangeal joints are flexed，a shape just like holding an egg. If the examinee can make a fist and extend fingers quickly，hand function is normal.

8-2-2　Joints of Lower Limbs

8-2-2-1　Hip Joints：The examinee lies on his/her back. The examiner presses the iliac crest with one hand and pushes the flexion knee joint to the chest with the other hand. The normal hip joint can flex 130°-140°. The examinee lies prone，the examiner presses the hip with one hand and holds the lower leg with the other hand. Bend the knee 90° and lift it up. The normal extension is 15°-30°. The examinee takes a supine position with his lower limbs straight and flat. The nurse moves one lower limb from the neutral position across the other lower limb to the opposite side. The normal adduction is 20°-30°. Move one side of the lower limb outward

骼相连，而背部的皮肤很薄，可以活动，因此手指可以弯曲。淋巴组织位于手背，这是在手部炎症的情况下，手背比手掌肿胀得更明显的原因。

手的功能位置是手腕背伸30°，尺偏15°，拇指外展，与指腹相对，近端指间关节弯曲，形状像拿着鸡蛋。如果受检者能够握拳并快速伸出手指，则手的功能正常。

8-2-2　下肢关节

8-2-2-1　髋关节：受检者仰卧，评估者一手按压其髂嵴，另一手将屈曲的膝关节推向前胸，正常髋关节可屈曲130°～140°；受检者俯卧，评估者一手按压臀部，另一手握小腿下端，屈膝90°后上提，正常可后伸15°～30°。受检者仰卧，双下肢伸直平放，护士将一侧下肢自中立位越过另一侧下肢向对侧活动，正常内收为20°～30°；将一侧下肢自中立位外移，远离躯体中线，正常外展为30°～45°。

from the neutral position, away from the midline of the body, and the normal abduction is 30°-45°. Keep the examinee's lower limbs straight and the patella and toe upward. The examiner's hands are placed under the examinee's thigh and knee to rotate the thigh, or the examinee bends the hip and knee to rotate the lower limbs inward or outward. The hip joint can be rotated inward or outward by 45°.

8-2-2-2　Knees: Try to flex the examinee's knee joint slowly, and the knee joint can flex 120°-150° normally. The examiner holds the examinee's knee and ankle and tries to straighten the knee from the flexion position. Under normal circumstances, the knee joint can be completely straightened, and sometimes there can be 5°-10° hyperextension.

The examinee keeps in supine position, with lower limbs relaxed. The examiner places the thumb of one hand apart from other four fingers on the top of the knee. Then, the examiner compresses the suprapatellar bursa to keep the fluid behind the patella. The other hand's thumb and middle finger fix below the joint, the index finger lightly presses the patella. If the joint cavity effusion is more than 50 mL, the patella will float up when press down and lift the index finger, which is indicated as the positive floating patella test.

保持受检者下肢伸直,髌骨和足尖向上,评估者将双手置于受检者大腿下部和膝部,旋转大腿,或受检者屈髋屈膝,向内侧或外侧转动下肢,髋关节可内旋或外旋 45°。

8-2-2-2　膝关节:缓慢地尽力屈曲受检者的膝关节,正常膝关节可屈曲 120°～150°。评估者握住患者的膝和踝关节,从屈曲位尽力伸直膝关节。正常情况下,膝关节能完全伸直,有时可有 5°～10°的过伸。

受检者取仰卧位,下肢放松。评估者将一手拇指与其余四指分开放置于膝关节上方,挤压髌上囊,将关节液积聚于髌骨后方,另一手拇指和中指固定在关节的下方,食指轻压髌骨。如关节腔积液超过 50 mL,则下压后松开食指可见髌骨向上浮起,称为浮髌试验阳性。

QR code 8-2-2-2　Floating patella test

二维码 8-2-2-2　浮髌试验

8-2-2-3　Ankles and Feet：Hold the examinee's foot and push it upward and downward，with normal back extension of 20°-30° and plantar flexion of 40°-50°. The examiner holds the examinee's ankle with one hand and the examinee's foot with the other hand，and moves the ankle to the left and right sides. The normal varus and valgus of the foot are 30° respectively.

Ask the examinee to straighten each toe, and then perform flexion and back extension. The normal plantar flexion is 30°-40° and back extension is 45°.

8-2-2-3　踝关节和足：握住受检者的足部，并将之向上方和下方推动，正常背伸 20°～30°，跖屈 40°～50°。评估者一手握住受检者的踝部，另一手握住受检者的足部并将踝部向左右两侧活动，正常足内、外翻各为 30°。

嘱受检者伸直各趾，然后做屈曲和背伸动作，正常跖屈 30°～40°，背伸 45°。

Words and Expressions

abduction　*n.* 外展

acromioclavicular　*n.* 肩锁关节

adduction　*n.* 引证，内收

ankle　*n.* 踝

arthritis　*n.* 关节炎

asymmetry　*n.* 不对称

bursa　*n.* 囊，黏液囊

cervical lordosis　颈椎前凸

dorsal extension　背伸

dorsum　*n.* 背（部）

elbow　*n.* 肘

epicondyles　*n.* 上髁

extension　*n.* 扩大,延伸,后伸

flexion　*n.* 弯曲,屈曲,前屈

hip　*n.* 髋

humeral　*adj.* 肱骨的

hyperemia　*n.* 充血

hypothenar　*n.* 小鱼际　*adj.* 小鱼际的

interspinous　*adj.* 椎间的,棘突间的

knee　*n.* 膝

lateral flexion　侧弯

ligament　*n.* 韧带

limb　*n.* 肢体,臂,腿

lumbar lordosis　腰椎前凸

olecranon　*n.* 鹰嘴

palmar flexion　掌屈

paravertebral　*adj.* 脊柱旁的,椎旁的

patella　*n.* 髌骨

proximal　*adj.* 近端的,近身体中心的

referred pain　放射痛

sacral kyphosis　尾椎后凸

scapula　*n.* 肩胛(骨)

sternoclavicular　*n.* 胸锁关节

suprapatellar　*adj.* 髌骨上的

thigh　*n.* 大腿,股部

thoracic kyphosis　胸椎后凸

varus　*n.* 内翻,弓形腿

valgus　*n. adj.* 外翻(的),外翻足

vertebral column　脊柱

visceral　*adj.* 内脏的,脏腑的

wrist　*n.* 手腕,腕关节

Assessment Skill 9
Neurological Assessment

评估技能 9
神经系统评估

The neurological assessment includes the following items: the assessment of cranial nerves, sensory function, motor function, neurological reflex, and autonomic function. Part of sensory function, motor function, and neurological reflex will be discussed here.

神经系统的评估包括脑神经检查、感觉功能评估、运动功能评估、神经反射评估和自主神经功能评估。这里主要介绍部分感觉功能评估、运动功能评估和神经反射评估。

9-1 Assessment of Sensory Function

9-1 感觉功能评估

Some basic principles should be kept in mind before starting sensory assessment. a. The examinees should remain alert and examiner needs to explain about why and how to do the sensory tests; b. a quiet environment is required for better feeling of different sensation; c. ask the examinee to close their eyes to avoid visual clues; d. start from the lesion site to the normal, compare the

感觉功能的检查需遵循以下原则：①受检者应保持警惕，评估者需要向受检者解释为什么，以及如何进行感觉测试；②环境安静；③要求受检者闭上眼睛，以避免出现视觉暗示；④从病变部位到正常部位，比较左右、上下、远端和近端的感

sensation between left and right，upper and down，distal and proximal part；e. when examining the examinees with consciousness impairment，examiner can only evaluate the sensation changes by judging the reaction of the examinee after sensory stimulation（e. g. painful facial expression，withdrawal limbs，etc.）.

9-1-1　Superficial Sensibility

9-1-1-1　Pain Sense：The examiner uses the tip of a pin to gently and evenly prickle the examinee's skin. Ask the examinee to state his or her feelings. Compare the bilateral feelings.

9-1-1-2　Touch：The examiner gently touches the examinee's torso or extremities skin with a cotton swab. Ask if the examinee feels the touch or not. Compare the bilateral feelings.

9-1-1-3　Temperature Sense：Two test tubes，one containing hot water（40-50 ℃）and the other containing cold water（5-10 ℃），are placed to contact with the skin of the examinee alternately. Let the examinee state his or her feelings. Compare the bilateral feelings.

9-1-2　Deep Sensation

9-1-2-1　Motor Sense：The examiner holds the fingers or toes of the examinee and keep them

觉;⑤当检查有意识障碍的受试者时,评估者只能通过判断受试者在感觉刺激后的反应来评估感觉变化(如痛苦的面部表情、四肢退缩等)。

9-1-1　浅感觉

9-1-1-1　痛觉:评估者用大头针的针尖均匀地轻刺受检者皮肤,让其陈述自己的感受,注意比较左右对称部位的感受。

9-1-1-2　触觉:评估者用棉签于左右对称部位轻触受检者躯干或四肢皮肤,询问受检者有无轻痒的感觉,注意比较左右对称部位的感受。

9-1-1-3　温度觉:分别用盛有热水(40～50 ℃)及冷水(5～10 ℃)的试管交替接触受检者皮肤,让其陈述自己的感受,注意比较左右对称部位的感受。

9-1-2　深感觉

9-1-2-1　运动觉:评估者用食指和拇指轻持受检

bent or stretched. Ask the examinee to answer "up" or "down" and check whether the answer is correct.

9-1-2-2　Posture Sense：The examiner places the limb of the examinee in a certain position to check whether he or she can accurately state the position of the limb，or let the examinee to imitate by the opposite limb.

9-1-2-3　Vibration Sense：The examiner uses a vibrating tuning fork to place on the bone hump of the examinee（such as medial malleolus，lateral malleolus，finger，radial ulnar styloid process，tibia，knee，etc.）and asks whether there is vibration.

9-2　Assessment of Motor Function

9-2-1　Assessment of Muscle Tension

The test for muscle tension is a passive movement.

9-2-1-1　Upper Limb Muscle Tension：The examinee keeps in supine position with muscles relaxed. The examiner touches the muscles of the upper arm and forearm respectively with both hands，and then the examinee performs passive elbow flexion and elbow extension，to sense the hardness of the muscles and the resistance during passive joint movement. Pay attention to bilateral comparison.

者的手指或足趾两侧做被动屈或伸的动作,让受检者回答"向上"或"向下",判断其回答是否正确。

9-1-2-2　位置觉:评估者将受检者的肢体放置在某种位置上,判断其是否能准确回答肢体所处的位置,或嘱其用对侧肢体模仿。

9-1-2-3　振动觉:评估者用震动的音叉放置在受检者的骨隆起处(如内踝、外踝、手指、桡尺骨茎突、胫骨、膝盖等),询问受检者有无振动感。

9-2　运动功能评估

9-2-1　肌张力评估

肌张力的检查是被动运动。

9-2-1-1　上肢肌张力:受检者仰卧,肌肉放松。评估者用双手分别触摸受检者上臂和前臂肌肉,再分别做被动屈肘和伸肘动作,感知受检者肌肉的硬度和关节被动运动时的阻力。注意双侧对比。

9-2-1-2 Lower Limb Muscle Tension: The examinee keeps in supine position with muscles relaxed. The examiner touches the muscles of thigh and calf muscles respectively with both hands, then the examinee performs passive knee flexion and knee extension, to sense the hardness of the muscles and the resistance during passive joint movement. Pay attention to bilateral comparison.

9-2-2 Assessment of Muscle Power

The test of muscle power is an active movement.

9-2-2-1 Upper Limb Muscle Power: Let the examinee bend and stretch the elbow actively, and the examiner resists from opposite directions to test the muscle power of the upper limb. The 0-5 grading method is used for evaluation. Pay attention to bilateral comparison.

Let the examinee clench the examiner's index finger and middle finger tightly. The examiner pulls them back hard to measure hand grip power. The 0-5 grading method is used for evaluation. Pay attention to bilateral comparison.

9-2-2-2 Lower Limb Muscle Power: Let the examinee bend and stretch the knee actively, and the examiner resists from opposite directions to test the muscle power of the lower limb. The 0-5 grading method is used for evaluation. Pay attention to bilateral comparison.

9-2-1-2 下肢肌张力:受检者仰卧,肌肉放松。评估者用双手分别触摸受检者大腿和小腿肌肉,再分别做被动屈膝和伸膝动作,感知受检者肌肉的硬度和关节被动运动时所受的阻力。注意双侧对比。

9-2-2 肌力评估

肌力的检查是主动运动。

9-2-2-1 上肢肌力:请受检者做主动曲肘和伸肘动作,评估者分别从相反的方向施加阻力,以测试其上肢肌力,采用0~5级评分法进行评价,注意双侧对比。

请受检者握紧评估者的食指和中指,评估者用力回抽以测试其手部握力,采用0~5级评分法进行评价,注意双侧对比。

9-2-2-2 下肢肌力:请受检者做主动屈膝和伸膝动作,评估者分别从相反的方向施加阻力以测试其下肢肌力,采用0~5级评分法进行评价,注意双侧对比。

QR code 9-2-2　Assessment of muscle power

二维码 9-2-2　肌力评估

9-2-3　Assessment of Coordinate Movement

9-2-3-1　Finger-to-nose Test：Ask the examinee to keep one upper limb straight and abducted, index finger straight and other four fingers close together. Then touch the tip of his nose repeatedly with the index finger, slowly first and then quickly. Pay attention to the comparison between eyes open and eyes closed, as well as the bilateral comparison. If the performance is not accurate, it may indicate ataxia.

9-2-3-2　Heel-knee-shin Test：The examinee keeps in supine position, straightens the left leg, and places the right heel on the left knee. Then, ask him/her to keep the right heel row down along the front of the shin. Notice whether the way of the heel is straight. If the heel action is unstable or wrong, it may indicate ataxia. Check the opposite side with the same method.

9-3　Assessment of Nerve Reflex

Neurological reflex evaluates the integrity of a local nerve circuit that consists of 5 components: sensory receptor, afferent

9-2-3　共济运动评估

9-2-3-1　指鼻试验：嘱受检者将一侧上肢伸直、外展，食指伸直，其余四指并拢，然后用伸直的食指反复触及自己的鼻尖，先慢后快。注意睁眼、闭眼及左右两侧的比较。如表现为指鼻不准，则提示可能有共济失调。

9-2-3-2　跟-膝-胫试验：受检者仰卧，将左侧下肢伸直，然后抬起右侧足跟置于左侧膝盖上，嘱其沿着胫骨前线向下划，注意观察足跟走向是否是直线。如足跟动作不稳或失误，则提示可能有共济失调。同法检查对侧。

9-3　神经反射评估

神经反射评估局部神经回路的完整性，其由 5 部分组成：感受器、传入神经、

nerve, nerve centre, efferent nerve and effector. It is usually less affected by the consciousness of the examinee but requires a considerate cooperation from the examinee. The examiner asks the examinee to be relaxed and compares the results between both sides as minor asymmetries can have a diagnostic significance. The major purpose of reflex examination is to differentiate central from peripheral nerve system lesions.

9-3-1 Superficial Reflex

Superficial reflex refers to the rapid muscle contraction reaction caused by stimulating skin, cornea and mucous membrane. In general, only unilateral superficial reflexes absence is considered abnormal, while bilateral absence often has no clinical diagnostic value.

9-3-1-1 Corneal Reflex: Ask the examinee to look inward and upward. The examiner gently touches the cornea with a fine cotton swab from the outside of the visual field to inward, avoiding touching the eyelashes. The normal response is the rapid closure of the stimulated eyelid, known as the direct corneal reflex; at the same time, the contralateral eyelid also closes, known as the indirect corneal reflex.

神经中枢、传出神经和效应器。它通常不受受检者意识的影响,但需要受检者全心配合。评估者嘱受检者放松,并对双侧的结果进行比较,因为轻微的不对称可能具有诊断意义。神经反射检查的主要目的是区分中枢神经系统和周围神经系统病变。

9-3-1 浅反射

浅反射是指刺激皮肤、角膜、黏膜所引起的肌肉急速收缩反应。通常情况下,单侧浅反射消失被认为是异常的,而双侧缺失往往没有临床诊断价值。

9-3-1-1 角膜反射:嘱受检者眼睛向内上方注视,评估者用细棉签纤维由视野外侧向内轻触受检者的角膜,注意避免触及睫毛。正常可见被刺激侧眼睑迅速闭合,称为直接角膜反射;同时对侧眼睑也出现闭合反应,称为间接角膜反射。

QR code 9-3-1-1　Corneal reflex

二维码 9-3-1-1　角膜反射

9-3-1-2　Abdominal Reflex：The examinee keeps in supine position with lower limbs slightly bent to relax the abdominal muscles. The examiner uses a cotton swab stick to gently scratch the abdominal wall skin from outside to inside in accordance with the three parts of the costal margin，the umbilicus and the groin. Normally，abdominal wall muscles contraction can be seen. Pay attention to bilateral comparison.

9-3-1-2　腹壁反射：受检者仰卧，双下肢稍曲以放松腹肌，评估者用棉签杆按照肋缘下、平脐、腹股沟三个部位由外向内轻轻划过腹壁皮肤，正常可见腹壁肌肉收缩，进行检查时注意左右对称。

QR code 9-3-1-2　Abdominal reflex

二维码 9-3-1-2　腹壁反射

9-3-1-3　Cremasteric Reflex：Ask the examinee to take supine position. Stroke the inner side of the thigh of the examinee from the bottom up(only men). The response is the elevation of the testicle on the stimulus side. Bilateral reflex absence of cremasteric reflex suggests ipsilateral cortical spinal tract lesions of lumber spinal L_{1-2}. Weakening or absence of unilateral reflex can be seen in pyramidal tract damage.

9-3-1-3　提睾反射：嘱患者仰卧，用棉签杆自下向上轻划股内侧上方皮肤（仅限男性受检者）。正常反应为同侧提睾肌收缩，睾丸上提；双侧反射消失见于腰髓1～2节病损；一侧反射减弱或消失见于锥体束损害。

9-3-1-4　Plantar Reflex：Ask the examinee to take supine position and put lower limbs straight. The examiner holds the examinee's ankle and strokes the sole along the lateral from the heel to the ball of the foot and then curve towards the big toe. The response is plantar flexion. The absence of plantar reflex indicates sacral spinal S_{1-2} dysfunction.

9-3-2　Deep Tendon Reflex

Deep tendon reflex refers to the rapid contraction reaction caused by the stimulation of tendons after sudden traction. Biceps reflex and triceps reflex in the upper limbs, patellar tendon reflex and achilles tendon reflex in the lower limbs are deep reflex.

9-3-2-1　Biceps Reflex：The examiner lifts the examinee's upper limb by the left arm，makes the examinee slightly bend the elbow and rotate the forearm inside. The examiner puts his/her left thumb on the biceps tendon and taps the left thumb with a percussion hammer in his/her right hand. The normal response is biceps contraction and rapid flexion of the forearm.

QR code 9-3-2-1　Biceps reflex

9-3-1-4　跖反射：嘱患者仰卧，双下肢伸直，护士手持患者踝部，用棉签杆沿足底外侧，由足跟向前划至小趾根部足掌时再转向踇趾侧。正常反应为足趾向跖面屈曲。反射消失见于骶髓1~2节病损。

9-3-2　深肌腱反射

深肌腱反射是指刺激肌腱突然受牵引后引起的急速收缩反应，包括上肢的肱二头肌反射和肱三头肌反射，下肢的膝腱反射和跟腱反射。

9-3-2-1　肱二头肌反射：评估者用左手臂托起受检者上肢，使其肘部稍弯曲，前臂稍内旋，评估者以左手拇指置于受检者肱二头肌肌腱上，右手持叩诊锤叩击左手拇指。正常反应为肱二头肌收缩，前臂呈现快速的屈曲动作。

二维码 9-3-2-1　肱二头肌反射

9-3-2-2　　Triceps Reflex：The examiner lifts the examinee's forearm and elbow by the left arm，flexes the elbow，rotates the forearm inside，and taps the triceps tendon above the olecranon with a percussion hammer in the right hand. The normal response is a contraction of the triceps and a slight extension of the forearm.

QR code 9-3-2-2　　Triceps reflex

9-3-2-3　　Patellar Tendon Reflex：The examinee keeps in the sitting position，with the legs drooping naturally，or keeps in supine position，while the examiner using the left hand to hold the upper area of the knee joint. The examiner's right hand holds a percussion hammer to tap the quadriceps tendon below the patella of the examinee. The normal response is quadriceps contraction and calf extension.

QR code 9-3-2-3　　Patellar tendon reflex

9-3-2-4　　Achilles Tendon Reflex：The examinee keeps in supine position with hips and knees flexed slightly，the lower limbs in

9-3-2-2　　肱三头肌反射：评估者用左手臂托起受检者前臂及肘关节，使其肘部屈曲、前臂内旋，右手持叩诊锤叩击受检者鹰嘴上方的肱三头肌肌腱。正常反应为肱三头肌收缩，前臂稍伸展。

二维码 9-3-2-2　　肱三头肌反射

9-3-2-3　　膝腱反射：受检者取坐位，小腿自然下垂，或取卧位。评估者用左手扶住受检者膝关节上方，右手持叩诊锤叩击受检者髌骨下方的股四头肌肌腱。正常反应为股四头肌收缩，小腿伸展。

二维码 9-3-2-3　　膝腱反射

9-3-2-4　　跟腱反射：受检者取仰卧位，髋、膝关节稍屈曲，下肢处于外展、外

abduction and external rotation. The examiner lifts the sole of the examinee's foot with his/her left hand，making the foot in over extension position，and taps the Achilles tendon with a percussion hammer in the examiner's right hand. The normal response is contraction of the gastrocnemius muscle and flexion of the foot towards the plantar.

旋位,评估者用左手托起受检者足底,使足呈过伸位,右手持叩诊锤叩击受检者跟腱。正常反应为腓肠肌收缩,足向跖面屈曲。

QR code 9-3-2-4　Achilles tendon reflex

二维码 9-3-2-4　跟腱反射

9-3-3　Abnormal Reflex

In the situation of pyramidal tract disease and in shock，coma，anesthesia，the brain loses the inhibitory effect on the brain stem and spinal cord，and the abnormal reflex is present，which is called pathological reflex，or positive pyramidal tract sign.

9-3-3-1　Babinski's Sign：The examinee keeps in supine position with lower limbs extended. The examiner holds the examinee's ankle in his/her left hand，and uses the cotton swab with the right hand to scratch forward along the outside of sole of foot to heel of small plantar and then turn to thumb. The normal reaction is the flexion of the toe to the metatarsal plane. If the thumb acts dorsal extension，and the other four toes act fan-shaped expansion，

9-3-3　病理反射

当受检者发生锥体束病损,以及在其休克、昏迷、麻醉时,大脑失去了对脑干和脊髓的抑制作用,而出现的异常反射,称为病理反射,也称锥体束征阳性。

9-3-3-1　巴宾斯基征:受检者仰卧,双下肢伸直,评估者左手持受检者脚踝,右手用棉签杆沿着受检者足底外侧向前划至小脚趾根部再转向姆趾。正常反应为足趾向跖面屈曲,如姆趾背伸,其余四趾呈扇形展开,则为病理征阳性。

which is a positive pathological sign.

QR code 9-3-3-1　Babinski's sign

二维码 9-3-3-1　巴宾斯基征

9-3-3-2　Oppenheim's Sign：The examinee keeps in supine position. The examiner uses her thumb and index finger to push hard from top to bottom along the front edge of the examinee's tibia. The normal reaction is the same as Babinski's sign.

9-3-3-2　奥本海姆征：受检者仰卧，评估者用拇指和食指沿着受检者胫骨前缘用力自上向下推动。正常反应同巴宾斯基征。

QR code 9-3-3-2　Oppenheim's sign

二维码 9-3-3-2　奥本海姆征

9-3-3-3　Gordon's Sign：The examinee keeps in supine position. The examiner squeezes the examinee's gastrocnemius muscles with thumb and other fingers. The normal reaction is the same as Babinski's sign.

9-3-3-3　戈登征：受检者仰卧，评估者用拇指和其余四指用力挤捏受检者腓肠肌。正常反应同巴宾斯基征。

QR code 9-3-3-3　Gordon's sign

二维码 9-3-3-3　戈登征

9-3-3-4　Hoffmann's Sign：The examiner holds the examinee's forearm near the wrist joint with the left hand，and uses the index

9-3-3-4　霍夫曼征：评估者用左手握住受检者前臂近腕关节处，右手食指和

and the middle finger of the right hand to clamp the examinee's middle finger and to lift it slightly so that the wrist is slightly over extended. Then the examiner quickly scratches the examinee's middle fingernail with the right thumb. The positive reaction is mild palmar curvature of the other four fingers.

中指夹持受检者中指并将其稍向上提,使其腕部轻度过伸,然后评估者用右手拇指迅速弹刮受检者中指指甲。阳性反应为受检者其余四指轻度掌屈。

QR code 9-3-3-4　Hoffmann's sign

二维码 9-3-3-4　霍夫曼征

9-3-4　Meningeal Irritation Sign

Meningeal irritation sign is the expression of meningeal irritation，seen in various meningitis，subarachnoid hemorrhage，increased cerebrospinal fluid pressure，etc.

9-3-4-1　Neck Rigidity：The examinee keeps in supine position without pillow，with neck relaxed，both lower limbs straightened naturally. The examiner passively flexes the examinee's neck by lifting occipital area and fixes the chest with the right hand，and then test the resistance of his/her neck muscles. Normally，there isn't neck resistance，and the lower jaw can touch the anterior chest wall.

9-3-4　脑膜刺激征

脑膜刺激征是脑膜受激惹的表现,见于各种脑膜炎、蛛网膜下腔出血、脑脊液压力增高等。

9-3-4-1　颈强直:受检者去枕平卧,颈部放松,双下肢自然伸直。评估者左手托起受检者枕部,右手固定其胸部,使其做被动屈颈动作以测试其颈肌抵抗力。正常人颈部无抵抗,下颌可触及前胸壁。

QR code 9-3-4-1　　Neck rigidity

9-3-4-2　Brudzinski's Sign：The examinee keeps in supine position with neck relaxed，both lower limbs straightened naturally. The examiner flexes the examinee's neck by lifting occipital area with the left hand and fixes the chest with the right hand. The normal reaction is that the lower jaw can touch the anterior chest wall，and the hip and knee joints are not flexed. If there is reflex flexion of hip and knee joint，it is the positive meningeal stimulation sign.

QR code 9-3-4-2　Brudzinski's sign

9-3-4-3　Kernig's Sign：The examinee keeps in supine position with one lower limb straightened naturally. The examiner lifts the other lower limb to bend the hip and knee to a nearly right-angled position. The knee joint is fixed by the left hand and the calf is raised by the right hand. Normal people can extend the knee more than 135°. If the examinee appears resistance within 135°，and accompanied with pain and flexor spasm，it is the positive meningeal stimulation sign.

二维码 9-3-4-1　　颈强直

9-3-4-2　布鲁金斯基征：受检者仰卧，双下肢自然伸直。评估者左手托起受检者枕部，右手固定其胸部，做被动屈颈动作。正常人下颌可触及其前胸壁，同时髋、膝关节无屈曲。如髋、膝关节有反射性屈曲，则为脑膜刺激征阳性。

二维码 9-3-4-2　　布鲁金斯基征

9-3-4-3　克尼格征：受检者仰卧，一侧下肢自然伸直。评估者抬起其另一侧下肢，使其屈髋屈膝至近乎直角状态，左手固定受检者膝关节，右手抬高受检者小腿。正常人膝关节可伸135°以上，如受检者在135°以内出现抵抗并伴有屈肌痉挛或疼痛，则为脑膜刺激征阳性。

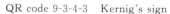

QR code 9-3-4-3　Kernig's sign

二维码 9-3-4-3　克尼格征

Words and Expressions

abdominal reflex　腹壁反射

Achilles tendon reflex　跟腱反射

afferent nerve　传入神经

autonomic function　自主神经功能

biceps reflex　肱二头肌反射

calf　*n.* 小腿

cerebrospinal fluid　脑脊液

corneal reflex　角膜反射

cremasteric reflex　提睾反射

deep reflex　深反射

direct corneal reflex　直接角膜反射

efferent nerve　传出神经

eyelash　*n.* 睫毛

eyelid　*n.* 眼睑

flexor spasm　屈肌痉挛

gastrocnemius muscles　腓肠肌

grip　*n. v.* 紧握, 紧抓

groin　*n.* 腹股沟

hammer　*n.* 锤子

indirect corneal reflex　间接角膜反射

ipsilateral cortical spinal tract　同侧皮质脊髓束

malleolus　*n.* 踝

meningeal irritation sign　脑膜刺激征

meningitis　*n*. 脑膜炎

metatarsal　*n*. 跖骨

motor function　运动功能

neurological　*adj*. 神经的

occipital　*adj*. 枕部的,枕骨的

patellar tendon reflex　膝腱反射

plantar reflex　跖反射

pyramidal tract　椎体束

quadriceps　*n*. 股四头肌

radial ulnar styloid process　桡尺骨茎突

sensory function　感觉功能

subarachnoid hemorrhage　蛛网膜下腔

superficial reflex　浅反射

tibia　*n*. 胫骨

triceps reflex　肱三头肌反射

Assessment Skill 10
Electrocardiography

操作技能 10
心电图描记法

QR code 10 Electrocardiography

二维码 10 心电图的描记

10-1 Preparation

10-1-1 Assessment

The examiner brings the ECG application form to the ward to check and assess the examinee.

10-1-2 Equipment Preparation

Prepare electrocardiograph, power cable, electrode cables, physiological saline, cotton swabs, bending plate and ECG paper.

10-1-3 Check the Electrocardiograph

Load the ECG paper into the

10-1 描记前准备

10-1-1 评估

检查者携心电图申请单至病房,核对并评估受检者。

10-1-2 用物准备

检查者准备心电图机、电源线、导联线、生理盐水、棉签、弯盘和心电图纸。

10-1-3 检测心电图机

检查者将心电图纸装

electrocardiograph, turn on and make sure it works well.

10-1-4　Examiner Preparation

Dress neatly and wash hands.

10-1-5　Check, Self Introduction and Explanation

Confirm the bed number and name of the examiner according to the ECG application form, introduce himself/herself to the examinee, ask the examinee to take off his/her watch, and ask him/her to breathe calmly and relax, and do not move during the recording process. If necessary, ask the examinee to hold the breath and record the chest lead ECG.

10-1-6　Environment Preparation

a. Close doors and windows, place screen if necessary, and keep the room warm to avoid cold stimulation; b. the examination bed should not be too narrow to ensure that the examinee lies comfortably, so as to avoid limbs tension; c. do not place other electrical appliances beside the examination bed; d. the power cord of the electrocardiograph should be as far away from the examination bed and the electrode cables as possible.

入心电图机,打开电源,确认机器状态完好。关机,去除电源线。

10-1-4　检查者准备

检查者须衣帽整齐、洗手。

10-1-5　核对、自我介绍与解释

按心电图申请单核对受检者床号、姓名,向受检者作自我介绍,嘱受检者取下手表,并嘱其在记录过程中平静呼吸并放松、不要移动四肢及躯体。必要时,需屏气记录胸导联心电图。

10-1-6　环境准备

①关闭门窗、必要时置屏风,保持室内温暖,以免寒冷刺激引起肌电干扰;②检查床不宜过窄,以保证受检者躺卧舒适,以免肢体紧张产生肌电干扰;③检查床旁不要摆放其他电器用具;④心电图机的电源线应尽可能远离检查床和导联电线。

10-2　ECG Record

10-2-1　Set up the Electrocardiograph

Turn on and input the information of examinee. Set the paper speed at 25 mm/s, calibration voltage at 10 mm/mV, press Anti Ac Interference key or Defibrillation Filter key if necessary.

10-2-2　Electrodes Placement

10-2-2-1　Limb leads：Expose the inside of both wrists and ankles. Apply physiological saline or conductive glue at about 3 cm above the wrists and about 7 cm above the ankles respectively. According to the electrode mark, place the limb lead electrode R（red）on the right wrist，L（yellow）on the left wrist，LF （green）on the left lower limb and RF（black） on the right lower limb.

10-2-2-2　Precordial lead：Undress the examinee's coat. After applying physiological saline to the examinee's chest V_1-V_6 respectively，place the chest lead at the corresponding part of V_1-V_6 according to lead electrodes of C_1-C_6. Red，yellow，green， brown，black and purple represent V_1-V_6 leads respectively.

10-2　描记心电图

10-2-1　设定心电图机

打开电源,输入受检者信息。设定走纸速度25 mm/s, 定标电压10 mm/mV,必要时按下抗交流电干扰键或去肌颤滤波键。

10-2-2　安置电极

10-2-2-1　肢体导联： 受检者暴露两手腕及脚踝, 分别在其左、右手腕曲侧腕关节上方约3 cm处,左、右脚踝上部约7 cm处涂上生理盐水或导电胶,按电极标记将肢体导联电极 R（红色）置于右手腕,L（黄色）置于左手腕,LF（绿色）置于左下肢, RF（黑色）置于右下肢。

10-2-2-2　心前区导联:解开受检者上衣,在受检者胸部 V_1～V_6 部位分别涂上生理盐水后,将胸导联与 C_1～C_6 对应,置于 V_1～V_6 相应的部位。红、黄、绿、褐、黑、紫分别代表 V_1～V_6导联。在心前区导联电极放置部位涂抹生理盐水后依次放置 V_1、 V_2、V_3、V_4、V_5 和 V_6导联。

V_1: The fourth intercostal space at the right edge of sternum.

V_2: The fourth intercostal space at the left edge of sternum.

V_4: The intersection of the left clavicular midline and the fifth intercostal.

V_3: The midpoint of the connecting line between V_2 and V_4.

V_5: The left axillary front line is at the same level as V_4.

V_6: The left axillary midline is at the same level as V_4.

10-2-3　Record ECG of Each Lead

Press the key to select the arrangement form of trace graphics. When the graphics are clear and the baseline is stable，ECG can be printed automatically or manually. If it is in automatic mode，the electrocardiograph will automatically print the ECG and then stop. In case of manual mode，after recording 3-5 ventricular waves，press the stop button to switch leads and record the ECG of other leads in turn.

Observe the reaction of the examinee during the operation. At the end of tracing，record the time.

V_1：胸骨右缘第 4 肋间。

V_2：胸骨左缘第 4 肋间。

V_4：左锁骨中线与第 5 肋间相交处。

V_3：V_2 与 V_4 两点连线中点。

V_5：左腋前线同 V_4 水平。

V_6：左腋中线同 V_4 水平。

10-2-3　描记各导联心电图

选择描记图形的排列形式,图形清晰、基线平稳,即可自动或手动采集心电图信号。如为自动模式,心电图机在采集完毕后自动停止并打印心电图;如为手动模式,在心电图机记录3～5 个心室波后,按下停止按钮,切换导联依次描记其余导联的心电图。

操作过程中注意观察受检者的反应,描记结束时,记录时间。

10-3　End of Tracing

10-3-1　Place Equipment

Turn off the electrocardiograph，tidy up the equipment.

10-3-2　Check the Examinee

Check the information of the examinee again. Tidy up the examinee.

10-3-3　Confirm the Information

Confirm the information on the ECG paper，such as the examinee's ward，bed number，examination time（year，month，day，hour，or even minute），the examiner's name，etc.

10-3-4　Mark Each Lead

Mark each lead correctly.

10-3　描记结束

10-3-1　归置用物

关闭心电图机，整理设备。

10-3-2　核对患者

再次核对受检者，并整理。

10-3-3　完善信息

在心电图纸上完善信息，如受检者所在病区、床号、检查时间（年、月、日、小时甚至分钟）、检查者姓名等。

10-3-4　标记各导联

正确标记各导联。

Simulated Case Study 1
Bronchial Asthma

模拟案例 1
支气管哮喘

Patient Wang Hong, female, 45 years old, farmer, primary school education level. Nationality: Han. Medical insurance: New Rural Cooperative Medical Insurance. Married, with a son of 23 years old. Her husband is 50 years old. The patient experienced expiratory dyspnea, was unable to lie flat and was with mobility restrictions. She coughed intermittently with a small amount of white frothy sputum. The patient was admitted to the inpatient department with diagnosis of 'bronchial asthma'.

Task: Please collect the patient's medical history, perform a specialized physical assessment for the patient, make nursing diagnoses based on previous information.

王红,女性,45 岁,农民,小学文化,汉族,新型农村合作医疗患者,已婚,儿子 23 岁,丈夫 50 岁。患者自觉呼气性呼吸困难,不能平卧,活动受限,间断咳嗽,咳少量白色泡沫样痰,门诊以"支气管哮喘"收住入院。

任务:请为患者采集病史;进行专科身体评估;按照评估内容提出该患者的护理诊断。

1. Medical History Collection

1.1 Key Points of Medical History Collection

1.1.1 General Information

The examiner introduces himself/herself to the patient.

General information of the patient: name, age, occupation, etc.

Medical coverage and payment method.

1.1.2 Main Symptoms

Name of main symptom: Expiratory dyspnea.

Inducing factors: Not found.

Degree of severity: Could not lie flat, with limited mobility.

1.1.3 Accompanying Symptoms

Accompanying symptom: Coughing and expectoration.

Characteristic: Coughing up white frothy sputa. Symptoms aggravating during night.

1.1.4 Diagnosis, Treatment and Nursing Process

This patient was diagnosed with asthma two years ago, while detailed information of the drug therapy was not provided.

1.1.5 Assessment of Daily Activities

Restricted mobility.

Poor sleep quality.

With normal diet and eats regularly, defecation and urination are all normal.

1. 病史采集

1.1 病史采集要点提示

1.1.1 一般项目

检查者自我介绍。

患者一般资料:姓名、年龄、职业等。

询问患者医疗费用支付形式。

1.1.2 主要症状

主要症状:呼气性呼吸困难。

诱因:无明显诱因。

程度:无法平卧;活动受限。

1.1.3 伴随症状

伴随症状:咳嗽咳痰。

伴随症状特点:咳白色泡沫样痰;咳嗽夜间加重。

1.1.4 诊断、治疗与护理经过

患者两年前被诊断为哮喘;曾用药治疗,具体成分不详。

1.1.5 日常生活状况

活动受限。

睡眠欠佳。

饮食、二便正常。

Living environment: Animals are raised at home.

1.1.6 Past Medical History

Denied the history of operation, hypertension, diabetes, etc.

History of allergy is unknown.

Born locally and not has been to epidemic areas before.

1.1.7 Family History

Patient's father has a history of asthma for 10 years.

Patient's mother, younger brother, husband and son are all healthy.

1.1.8 History of Marriage, Birth and Menstruation

Married and had a natural delivery.

With regular menstruation.

1.1.9 Psycho-Social Status

With anxiety.

With well-functioning economic and social supporting systems.

1.2 Cautions of Medical History Collection

1.2.1 Ask from general questions to specialized questions.

1.2.2 Avoid leading questions and multiple questions.

1.2.3 Ask in the order of scoring system.

1.2.4 Quote and confirm information provided by the patient.

家庭环境:饲养动物。

1.1.6 既往史

否认手术史、高血压、糖尿病等病史。

过敏史不详。

当地出生、未去过疫区。

1.1.7 家族史

父亲患哮喘 10 年。

母亲、弟弟、丈夫、儿子身体健康。

1.1.8 婚育史与月经史

适龄婚育、正常分娩。

月经正常。

1.1.9 心理社会情况

情绪焦虑。

经济及社会支持系统良好。

1.2 病史采集注意事项

1.2.1 提问遵循从一般到特殊的原则。

1.2.2 无诱导性提问，连续性提问。

1.2.3 按项目的问诊评分顺序系统提问。

1.2.4 引证核实患者提供的信息。

1.2.5 Pause and summarize during the history taking.

1.2.6 Listen attentively and do not interrupt unless necessary.

1.2.7 Avoid awkward pauses.

1.2.8 Communicate with amicable eye contact, proper body language and encouraging phrases.

1.2.9 Communicate with positive praise and encouragement.

1.2.10 Avoid questions with medical terms or jargons, if necessary, explanation should be provided.

1.2.11 Dress properly and behave in good manners. Develop a harmonious relationship with the patient.

1.2.12 Be modest and respect the patient. Try to build a relationship of mutual trust.

1.2.13 Be compassionate and give comfort to the patient.

1.2.14 Transitional and summarizing remarks are necessary during history taking.

2. Specialized Physical Assessment

2.1 Key Points of Specialized Physical Assessment

2.1.1 Materials and instruments preparation: therapeutic trolley, ruler, marker pen, stethoscope, hand sanitizer.

1.2.5 问诊过程中有小结。

1.2.6 询问者注意聆听,不轻易打断患者讲话。

1.2.7 不出现难堪的停顿。

1.2.8 给予患者友好的眼神,适当的体语以及鼓励的短语。

1.2.9 给予患者赞扬性肯定或鼓励。

1.2.10 不使用医学名词或术语提问,如果使用术语必须立即向患者解释。

1.2.11 衣冠整洁,举止端庄,建立与患者的和谐关系。

1.2.12 谦虚礼貌,尊重患者,获取患者的信任。

1.2.13 有同情心,使患者感到温暖。

1.2.14 问诊应有过渡语言及结束语。

2. 专科身体评估

2.1 专科身体评估内容提示

2.1.1 用物准备:治疗车,直尺,记号笔,听诊器,洗手液。

2.1.2 After washing hands, the examiner explains to the patient and properly exposes the chest of the patient.

2.1.3 Inspect the contour of the chest, the skin, the respiration movement (frequency, rhythm and depth).

2.1.4 Palpate thoracic expansion.

2.1.5 Palpate for vocal fremitus on both sides of chest wall.

2.1.6 Palpate to verify the existence of pleural friction.

2.1.7 Percuss anterior chest wall and lateral chest wall (on both sides).

2.1.8 Percuss the inferior boundary of lungs.

2.1.9 Auscultate anterior chest wall and lateral chest wall.

2.1.10 Auscultate vocal resonance on both sides of chest wall.

2.1.11 Auscultate pleural friction rub.

2.1.12 Expose the back, inspect the contour and skin.

2.1.13 Palpate mobility of chest wall and its symmetry.

2.1.14 Ask the patient to cross both arms and put hand on the opposite shoulder, upper body slightly leans forward.

2.1.15 Percuss the back.

2.1.16 Percuss the inferior boundary mobility of lungs and measure it.

2.1.17 Ask the patient to take a deep

2.1.2 检查者洗手后与患者交流,并正确暴露患者胸部。

2.1.3 视诊胸部外形、皮肤,呼吸运动的频率、节律、深度等。

2.1.4 触诊胸廓扩张度。

2.1.5 触诊双侧语音震颤。

2.1.6 触诊胸膜摩擦感。

2.1.7 叩诊双侧前胸和侧胸。

2.1.8 叩诊肺下界。

2.1.9 听诊双侧前胸和侧胸。

2.1.10 听诊双侧语音共振。

2.1.11 听诊胸膜摩擦音。

2.1.12 充分暴露背部,视诊背部外形、皮肤等。

2.1.13 触诊胸廓活动度及对称性。

2.1.14 嘱患者双上肢交叉,双手分别置于对侧肩部,身体稍前倾。

2.1.15 叩诊背部。

2.1.16 叩诊肺下界移动范围,并测量。

2.1.17 嘱患者深呼吸,

breath，then auscultate both sides of the lungs symmetrically.

2.2 Cautions of Specialized Physical Assessment

2.2.1 Examination should be based on the principles of local examination orders and in accordance with the order of the checklist. Examine with caution and prudence.

2.2.2 Examine with correct methods and proficiency.

2.2.3 Offer effective communication and protection to the patient.

3. Assessment and Diagnoses

Evaluate with role-playing method. Make nursing diagnoses based on data acquired above.

双侧对称地听诊肺部。

2.2 专科身体评估注意事项

2.2.1 遵照条目顺序及局部查体顺序的原则，认真仔细地检查。

2.2.2 手法正确规范、检查熟练。

2.2.3 注意与患者进行交流，注意保护患者。

3. 评估与诊断

按照角色扮演的方法进行评估，根据评估所获资料，提出该患者的护理诊断。

Simulated Case Study 2
Hypertension

模拟案例 2

高血压

Patient Li Lijun, male, 48 years old, worker, medical insurance: not covered. Married, with a daughter of 20 years old. His wife is 46 years old and is a worker. The patient felt dizzy and suffered from a headache, with blood pressure 180/100 mmHg, body temperature is normal, with expression of anxiety and flushed face. The patient complained of intermittent dizzy and headache for 3 years, the conditions worsened in the past 3 days. The patient was admitted to the inpatient department with diagnosis of 'hypertension'.

Vital signs: T 36.5 ℃; P 96 beats/min; R 20 times/min; BP 180/100 mmHg.

Task: Please collect medical history,

李力军,男性,48 岁,工人,无医保。已婚,妻子 46 岁,工人,女儿 20 岁。该患者头晕、头痛,血压 180/100 mmHg,体温正常,表情焦虑,颜面绯红;主诉间断性头晕头痛 3 年,近 3 天加重。门诊以"高血压"收住入院。

生命体征:T 36.5 ℃;P 96 次/分;R 20 次/分;BP 180/100 mmHg。

任务:请为患者采集病

perform a specialized physical assessment for the patient，make nursing diagnoses based on previous information.

史，进行专科身体评估，并根据评估所获资料提出该患者的护理诊断。

1. Medical History Collection

1. 病史采集

1.1 Key Points of Medical History Collection

1.1.1 The examiner introduces himself/herself to the patient.

1.1.2 General Information

Li Lijun，male，48 years old，worker，without any medical coverage. Married. His wife，who is also a worker，is in poor health status. Relationship between the couple is good. With a daughter of 20 years old，who will participate in the national college entrance exam soon. No religious belief.

1.1.3 Chief Complaint

Intermittent vertigo and headache for 3 years and has been worsening for 3 days.

1.1.4 Characteristics of Main Symptoms

Inducing factors：Medication was taken intermittently；tiredness，emotional disturbance，unhealthy diet.

Duration：2 hours for each attack.

Accompanying symptoms：Heart palpitations，tinnitus.

Method of alleviation：Rest.

1.1.5 Deterioration of Main Symptoms

Inducing factors：Suffered a headache

1.1 病史采集要点提示

1.1.1 检查者自我介绍

1.1.2 患者一般资料

李力军，男性，48 岁，工人，无医保。已婚，妻子 46 岁，体弱多病，工人，夫妻感情和睦。女儿 20 岁，马上面临高考。无宗教信仰。

1.1.3 主诉

间断性头晕头痛 3 年，近 3 天加重。

1.1.4 主要症状特点

诱因：间断服药，劳累，情绪激动，饮食不合理。

持续时间：每次 2 个小时。

伴随症状：心悸、耳鸣。

缓解：休息。

1.1.5 主要症状加重情况

诱因：跟邻居生了点气

after falling out with a neighbour.

Duration：3 days.

Alleviation：The symptoms did not alleviate.

Accompanying symptoms：Heart palpitations, tinnitus.

1.1.6 Diagnosis，Treatment and Nursing Process

History of medication：Has been taking anti-hypertensive drugs intermittently.

Treatment history：Was hospitalized for treatment 3 years ago.

1.1.7 Assessment of Daily Activities

Sleep quality, diet, defecation and urination.

Smoking history：Has been smoking for 20 years，20 cigarettes per day.

Alcohol intake history：20 years.

1.1.8 Past Medical History

With hypertension.

Without history of diabetes.

Without history of hyperlipidemia.

1.1.9 History of Marriage and Birth

Married and has a daughter.

1.1.10 Family History

Patient's father has a history of hypertension.

Patient's mother is in poor health status.

Patient's younger sister is healthy.

1.1.11 Psycho-Social Status

With anxiety.

Economic and social supporting systems are not sufficient.

后,感到头疼。

持续时间:3天。

缓解:不缓解。

伴随症状:心悸、耳鸣。

1.1.6 诊断治疗与护理经过

用药史:间断服用降压药。

治疗经过:3年前住院治疗。

1.1.7 日常生活状况

睡眠、饮食、二便。

吸烟史:20年,20支/天。

饮酒史:20年。

1.1.8 既往史

高血压病史。

无糖尿病病史。

无高脂血症病史。

1.1.9 婚育史

适龄婚育,育有一女。

1.1.10 家族史

父亲高血压病史。

母亲身体不好,妹妹体健。

1.1.11 心理社会情况

情绪焦虑。

经济与社会支持系统较差。

1.2 Cautions of Medical History Collection

1.2.1 Ask from general questions to specialized questions.

1.2.2 Avoid leading questions and multiple questions.

1.2.3 Ask in the order of scoring system.

1.2.4 Quote and confirm information provided by the patient.

1.2.5 Pause and summarize during the history taking.

1.2.6 Listen attentively and do not interrupt unless necessary.

1.2.7 Avoid awkward pauses.

1.2.8 Communicate with amicable eye contact, proper body language and encouraging phrases.

1.2.9 Communicate with positive praise and encouragement.

1.2.10 Avoid questions with medical terms or jargons, if necessary, explanation should be provided.

1.2.11 Dress properly and behave in good manners. Develop a harmonious relationship with the patient.

1.2.12 Be modest and respect the patient. Try to build a relationship of mutual trust.

1.2.13 Be compassionate and give comfort to the patient.

1.2 病史采集注意事项

1.2.1 从一般到特殊的提问。

1.2.2 无诱导性提问，连续性提问。

1.2.3 按项目的问诊评分顺序系统地问。

1.2.4 引证核实患者提供的信息。

1.2.5 问诊过程中有小结。

1.2.6 询问者注意聆听，不轻易打断患者讲话。

1.2.7 不出现难堪的停顿。

1.2.8 给予患者友好的眼神，适当的体语以及鼓励的短语。

1.2.9 给予赞扬性肯定或鼓励。

1.2.10 不使用医学名词或术语提问，如果使用术语必须立即向患者解释。

1.2.11 衣冠整洁，举止端庄，建立与患者的和谐关系。

1.2.12 谦虚礼貌，尊重患者，获得患者的信任。

1.2.13 有同情心，使患者感到温暖。

1.2.14 Transitional and summarizing remarks are necessary during the history taking.

2. Specialized Physical Assessment

2.1 Key Points of Specialized Physical Assessment

2.1.1 Materials and instruments preparation: therapeutic trolley, ruler, marker pen, stethoscope, hand sanitizer.

2.1.2 After washing hands, the examiner explains to the patient properly.

2.1.3 Inspect the eyelids and face for edema, inspect the mouth and lips for existence of cyanosis.

2.1.4 Inspect carotid arteries and jugular veins.

2.1.5 Expose the chest properly.

2.1.6 Inspect the precordium (prominence or depression, abnormal apex impulse, normal apex impulse).

2.1.7 Palpate the radial arteries on both sides.

2.1.8 Adopt the double-step method to palpate apex impulse.

2.1.9 Palpate to determine if there's fremitus or pericardial friction.

2.1.10 Auscultate breath sound on both lungs (at lung bases, to auscultate at least three pairs of places).

2.1.11 Percuss relative cardiac dullness

1.2.14 问诊应有过渡语言及结束语。

2.专科身体评估

2.1 专科身体评估内容提示

2.1.1 用物准备：包括治疗车，直尺，记号笔，听诊器，洗手液。

2.1.2 检查者洗手与患者交流。

2.1.3 视诊眼睑、颜面有无水肿，口唇有无发绀。

2.1.4 视诊颈动、静脉有无异常。

2.1.5 正确暴露胸部。

2.1.6 视诊心前区（有无隆起或凹陷、异常心尖搏动或正常心尖搏动）。

2.1.7 触诊双侧桡动脉。

2.1.8 两步法触诊心尖搏动。

2.1.9 触诊有无震颤，心包摩擦感。

2.1.10 听诊双肺呼吸音（至少 3 对，双肺底听诊）。

2.1.11 叩诊心脏相对

(left border).

2.1.12 Percuss relative cardiac dullness (right border).

2.1.13 Auscultate the apical area (heart rate and heart rhythm).

2.1.14 Auscultate the valve areas.

2.1.15 Examine if the hepato jugular reflux sign is positive.

2.1.16 Palpate both lower limbs for edema.

2.1.17 Palpate the dorsalis pedis arteries on both sides.

2.2 Cautions of Specialized Physical Assessment

2.2.1 Examination should be based on the principles of local examination orders and in accordance with the order of the checklist. Examine with caution and prudence.

2.2.2 Examine with correct methods and proficiency.

2.2.3 Offer effective communication and protection to the patient.

3. Assessment and Diagnoses

Evaluate with role-playing method. Make nursing diagnoses based on data acquired above.

浊音界(左界)。

2.1.12 叩诊心脏相对浊音界(右界)。

2.1.13 心尖区听诊(心率、心律)。

2.1.14 各瓣膜区听诊。

2.1.15 检查肝颈回流征是否为阳性。

2.1.16 触诊双下肢有无水肿。

2.1.17 触诊双侧足背动脉。

2.2 专科身体评估注意事项

2.2.1 遵照条目顺序及局部查体顺序的原则,认真仔细地检查。

2.2.2 手法正确规范、检查熟练。

2.2.3 注意与患者进行交流,注意保护患者。

3.评估与诊断

按照角色扮演的方法进行资料的收集,按照收集到的资料提出该患者的护理诊断。

References

参考文献

[1]FENSKE C，WATKINS K，SAUNDERS T，et al. Health & physical assessment in nursing [M]. 4th ed. New Jersey：Pearson Education，Inc，2020.

[2]万学红. Chinical diagnostics[M]. 北京：人民卫生出版社，2017.

[3]孙玉梅,张立力. 健康评估(第 4 版)[M]. 北京：人民卫生出版社,2017.